TIME TO SUCCEED
ACTION GOALS FOR WEIGHT LOSS

BY

HOLLY ALASTRA, RD, LCPC, Weight Management Expert

&

JASON WILCOX, LCSW, Life and Corporate Coach

GRAY BEACH PUBLISHING

TIME TO SUCCEED
ACTION GOALS FOR WEIGHT LOSS

Gray Beach Publishing
2016

First Paperback Edition: 2014

Holly Alastra & Jason Wilcox
Time To Succeed: Action Goals For Weight Loss

ISBN: **978-1540681126**

Cover design by Jason Wilcox

Printed in the United States of America

CHAPTER ONE

Action Goals

Here is a quick suggestion before you begin this book. While you read, make sure to have paper and pen close by to write down thoughts and ideas that come to mind. These notes will play a powerful part in your success and Action Goal development.

Importance of Action Goals. Your life is an accumulation of the choices you've made, what you have or haven't done. Have you ever had that moment where you look around and ask yourself, "What the heck am I doing here?" Maybe this question applies to your job, relationship, health, weight, or any other life situation. These moments are golden opportunities in life because once you question your situation, you are going to make a choice. Some people make the choice to take steps towards change, while others may decide to keep the status quo.

Now, you can't change the past, so there's no use dwelling on it. However, you can learn from the past and make choices today that are in alignment with the person you want to be and the life you want to live. You have more power in creating the life you desire than you may realize.

Your thoughts become your reality, and having the thought, 'It's time to make a change,' is a tremendous leap into living your best life.

Throughout this book we are going to talk about some of the most important steps to success in living your best life. One of the most critical elements to creating this success are Action Goals. Properly set Action Goals can change a choice from a thought to a reality. We will help you design effective goals to help you lose weight. . "What can I do today?" will be a key question to ask yourself throughout this book.

So, shall we begin? Let's talk about Action Goals.

"Goals?" Some of you may be asking. Maybe you've already been down this road. You've set goals in the past and haven't achieved them, so why bother? Well don't close the book quite yet. There are reasons why some of you may not have succeeded with your goals in the past. When a goal doesn't work out, it's a very frustrating and deflating feeling. This time can be different. We'll outline what makes a successful goal and what doesn't. You can achieve your goals and feel the inspiring confidence that comes with accomplishment.

Action Goals are the tools that give good choices the strength to happen. Whether individuals recognize they are engaged in Action Goals or not, they are at the heart of any great accomplishment.

Let's take a rock climber, for example. In order to make it to the top of the cliff there's going to be some very specific and realistic steps (Action Goals) that the climber will use to be successful. Without them the climber won't make it to the top.

Outcome vs. Goal. Many things can get in the way of goals, you know, like goalies. However, we aren't talking about soccer here, we're talking about Action Goals. We have found that the biggest thing that keeps people from achieving their goals isn't what you might think. It's actually the fact that a lot of people set outcomes as their goals. If you set an outcome, which is an end result, for your Action Goal, you dramatically decrease your chance for success, and it may feel like a professional goalie actually is blocking every attempt you make.

Let's say you want to lose weight and your goal is to lose five pounds over the next week or two. You have set a desired outcome as your Action Goal. Losing the weight isn't something you can do, it's a result that comes after taking actions, or in other words, completing Action Goals. So an Action Goal would look more like walking for thirty minutes a day. That, my friends, is something you can do. It's an action that you can start today. This is the very core of an Action Goal. When you set an Action Goal one of the key questions you need to ask yourself is, "Does my Action Goal have actual steps I can start today or this week?"

Again, Action Goals lead to outcomes, but Action Goals are not the same as your desired outcomes. A desired outcome is getting to the top of the cliff you're climbing. The Action Goals are grabbing ahold of the rock face, getting your foothold, securing your rope, and moving up the cliff side. Without these steps, you'll never reach the outcome of getting to the top of the cliff, or in other words, losing the weight that you want to lose.

One of Jason's clients, Samantha, is a great example of this. Years ago, and some time after she married, she set what she felt to be a simple goal: lose weight. But like so many people trying to lose weight, she found herself feeling frustrated at every turn, and was not succeeding in her goal. However, as she stopped focusing so intensely on her goal (which was actually an outcome), and focused on very specific Action Goals to modify her diet and physical activity levels, she began to see results. When she was solely focused on the outcome that she couldn't directly control, she found herself stuck and at times moving backwards, which led her to feel disheartened and upset. Often times so much so that she considered giving up.

To understand why she was ready to give up, let's look at the cliff climbing metaphor. If the climber is solely focused on the outcome or making it to the top of the cliff, then the climber is going to be constantly making mistakes, not focused on where she is putting her hands, feet, and rope. She might end up slipping or falling, and possibly even getting seriously hurt.

The other reason it can be discouraging has to do with the perception that the end outcome never seems to get closer when we are so focused on it. Remember those days in the boring class at school when you watched the clock and time seemed to take forever? You felt stuck. The same principle applies when we get so focused on the outcome; we get stuck and can't take the steps we need to take to ever arrive at our ultimate aspiration.

As Samantha discovered, it's better to set the outcome and then put it to the side. You need to know where you are going, but once you've set the outcome, it becomes important to stop focusing on it and turn your full attention to your Action Goals and what you're doing in the moment or that day. When you do so, you'll feel the traction and momentum from your success and accomplishments, and will be more likely to shake off any setbacks and the accompanying feelings of discouragement.

Share Your Success and Accomplishments.

"I'm going to start working out on my elliptical machine again."

"As soon as the weather is nicer, I'm going to start walking."

"Starting tomorrow, I'm going to eat better."

Can you identify with the types of thoughts above? People have thoughts like these all the time—and nothing happens. We've all been there. Sometimes our thoughts don't turn into actions. Especially when it comes to exercise and eating healthy.

Throughout this book, there are lots of ideas to make your thoughts turn into action. One critical step you can take is to tell someone your Action Goals. You may think that it's better to keep your goals to yourself just in case you aren't successful. But finding the right person to confide in can actually help you succeed. Who will be supportive and excited for you when you accomplish your goals? Aim to find at least one person: maybe a sibling, a parent, a spouse, or a friend. Once you've identified your support person or persons, let them know your goals and ask for their support. You might ask to check in with them daily to share your successes or failures. If you do not succeed, your support person can act as a sounding board to help you come up with ideas that will help you do better next time. Even better yet, see if you can find someone who also wants to set their own Action Goals, and you can share your progress with one another.

On the follow-up goals page, you have spaces you can fill in to show what you were able to accomplish. This is a great visual for you to see the successes you are having. We also suggest that you show others your follow-up goals pages. If you are struggling you can let them know what you're struggling with, and they might have some great ideas on what might work to help get you over the hump so you can reach your success. If you are working on goals together, try to generate ideas for your support person to help them overcome any areas where they may be struggling as well.

Your successes will increase if you have someone that you can check in with each week, and they will probably feel excited about helping you. Just think about it. How would you feel if someone close to you approached you and said, "Would you be willing to help me out with a few goals?" or "Could I check in with you each week and tell you about everything I was able to accomplish?" It would probably make you feel good that someone would trust you in such a significant part of their life.

Now, don't stop with just telling your support person the Action Goal. Make sure to follow up and tell them about your progress on a daily or at least weekly basis. Tell them about your accomplishments, even if these accomplishments only resulted from a "learning" moment when you didn't succeed. Be excited about what you accomplish every week and bring others into the exciting world with you. Enthusiasm is key because it helps keep us going even during hard times when we want to just give up.

Make it Fun. There is nothing like trying to get yourself to do something you hate. Years ago Jason's client, Samantha, used to bug her husband about getting a joint gym membership. He told her that he didn't really care for working out in gyms. He isn't much of a social exerciser, to put it mildly. However, after a year of listening to her request that they join the gym, he gave in.

The next few months, she had a great time going to the gym and working out. He was miserable. It truly was torture for him, but he did his best to be a supportive husband and stuck with it for a while. When the day came that they decided to end the membership, he did his best to hold back his excitement, but boy he was a happy man. The problem was simple, he hated going to the gym to work out. He enjoyed peaceful runs in the country or just working out at the house. Trying to make himself enjoy working out at the gym was a dead-end game.

When setting goals, you want to make sure you find things that you might enjoy or at minimum find something you don't distain. If you don't like running, try to find something you like to do. Get creative. Go hiking, play a sport, play your Wii fit or Xbox Kinect, go dancing, take a class, etc. You can also couple physical activity with something you enjoy. Watch a show, listen to your favorite music, or even try a book on CD while you run on the treadmill or workout. The same goes for diet. Experiment with recipes and find tasty ways to eat fruits and vegetables, such as in smoothies, salads, or stir-fry. The sky is the limit. Involve others and share your creative and healthy recipes. It feels great when friends and family get excited about your healthy creations. But the point is you can succeed without eating something you don't like or doing something you don't like. Healthy food can and should taste good. Exercise can be fun.

Are you thinking about what might be enjoyable for you? Make sure to write down all of the ideas that pop into your mind, and then include them in your Action Goals.

Other ways to make things fun includes: adding rewards if you achieve your goals, compete against others, or engage in healthy activities with friends and loved ones. Rewards could be anything you like to do or might save up to buy. Jason loves fishing, so he sets his goals and if he completes them, he gets to go on a fishing trip. Make a list of rewards that would help entice you to succeed in your goals. Friendly competitions can turn a monotonous task into a lot of fun. You might have a points chart for you and whomever you are competing with, or you can compete with time exercised, distance walked, biked, or ran, number of servings of vegetables eaten daily, etc.

Growing up, Jason and his brother had competitions with eating vegetables that they didn't like. Neither of them liked radishes or tomatoes. So, one day they competed to see who could eat the most tomatoes. Lets just say Jason won and hopes his brother isn't reading this book. But we both ate our share of tomatoes that day!

If you use the chart idea, you can use an online program or you can literally post a chart in the house to write down your score. Posting something for everyone to see also gets others involved in your goals, which is hugely important, as we discussed before. Jason and his wife have a chart in their room that they use to mark the time they exercise every week. Who ever has the most points by the time of their next date gets to pick what they do on the date. This helps keep things fun, gives them a reward, tracks what they've done, and keeps them accountable to one another. These are all important elements in helping them keep their goals and will be for you as well.

Remember, if you set an Action Goal that you really hate, you're taking something that's already tough and turning it into something almost impossible. Why make something harder than it needs to be? Find a way to make it enjoyable.

Triggers For Success. Our lives are often busy, filled with work, obligations, activities, and the list goes on and on. With the demands each of us faces in the modern-day world, it's tough to squeeze in lifestyle changes. On top of that, whenever we repeat something over and over, the brain forms neural pathways that get stronger and stronger, meaning that if we try to change our habits, we actually have to rewire our brain. The neural pathway becomes a well-worn road that holds deep ruts. They can be difficult to get out of. However, the good news is that, over time, good habits can become just as engrained as bad habits. You can begin to create a very strong path in your brain that will guide you to healthy behaviors.

A few years ago Jason's client, Steven, made a decision he was going to start working out in the mornings. It lasted a few days, but not too long. The same thing happened when he decided he would workout right after work. After about a week of coming home and changing into gym clothes, he threw in the towel. Then he came up with the idea of ideas. He would workout at lunchtime. Can you guess what happened? You're right, it didn't last. He always became too involved with work to take time to workout.

His normal life routine, or habit, was to sleep until it was time to go to work in the morning, plow through work rather than take a break midday, and do housework after work, so when he added something new into his routine it was difficult for him to keep the new routine. We often follow the path of least resistance. This path of least resistance is whatever our daily habits happen to be. Steven used to get up in the morning, get ready for work, work all day, return home, eat dinner, watch his favorite shows on TV, and get ready for bed. Think of your daily routine as a path that you walk each day. It is hard to venture off of our favorite, well-worn, path, and sometimes we need something to help totally knock us off this path. What can push us onto a new, better path, and one that will ultimately be more fulfilling? A trigger.

A trigger is a daily activity that can help push you out of your routine. For example, one individual Jason had been working with tried multiple ways to get herself to start doing more physical activity. Despite her attempts, she was unsuccessful until she came up with a brilliant idea to start taking walks every time she used the restroom—not long walks, just up and down the hallways and stairs for about five minutes. However, it helped her each day to get her walking goal accomplished. Each week she added a couple of minutes to her walking time. She began to lose weight, and she felt great about her success.

Try to think of something that can initiate a change in your routine or interrupt your habits. Something that pulls you away can be very effective. Maybe you decide to take a drink of water whenever you get a text message. Maybe you commit to doing strength training during your favorite TV show. Maybe after the TV show you get up and make yourself a healthy lunch with fruit and vegetables for the next day.

Other ideas that might interrupt your routine are: an alarm on your phone, planning to go for a walk after you finish the dishes, packing a gym bag and driving straight to the gym after work rather than going home first, or planning to meet a friend for an early morning workout.

Your Action Goal Chart. Before you get started, there is a sample Action Goal chart on the next page to help you get an idea of what a specific action goal looks like. Your Action Goal journal will start after Chapter Two.

Date: _9/29_

Desired Outcome: _I want to lose 20 lbs_

Specific Action: _Ride my exercise bike for 45 minutes_

When will you start: _Tomorrow Morning_

What Days and Times? _Mon, Wed, Fri In the morning before I go to Work_

How will you accomplish? _First thing in the morning before anything else_

What do you need? _Exercise bike._

How will you make it fun? _Watch my favorite shows while I work out._

Who do you tell? _My spouse, and my two closest friends._

What will get in your way? _If I don't get enough sleep it will be hard to get up in time._

How will you overcome challenges? _Set an alarm on my phone to make sure I go to bed early enough_

CHAPTER TWO

STEPS FOR SUCCESSFUL ACTION GOALS

Good vs. Bad. Many of us were raised with the idea of good and bad, black and white, right and wrong. What would happen if you stepped away from those ideas while working on your goals? Now we're not suggesting that you get rid of accountability or values. On the contrary, we're suggesting making a commitment not to judge yourself as you go through this process. Accountability is a very important piece, but it can be done without judgments.

Let's take a look at a few real-life situations that highlight how judgments can get in the way of success. A good friend of Jason's came to him a few years ago very upset. She looked around at actresses and others who were able to lose weight quickly after having children. In her mind, it was unacceptable that she wasn't in better shape. She felt like a failure because she was still overweight despite her attempts to shed the pounds. We'll address the mythical "failure" part a little later.

For now, we can tell you that she coped with her anger and sadness over not being thinner by turning to food to help her feel better, which in turn prevented her from losing weight, and then made her feel worse. It was a vicious cycle.

In another situation, a gentleman Jason worked with struggled to stick with his goals because he set unrealistic ones. Starting out, this man expected himself to be capable of far more than was physically possible at his level of fitness. He thought he should be able to go out and run a marathon, and because he couldn't, he didn't see the point of even trying. He needed to start with something more doable, possibly small walks and light weights. Though he viewed this level of activity as pathetic, over time, he learned that nobody starts out on top. Anybody who excels starts at the bottom and spends countless hours practicing. Jason's client began to set more achievable goals, and this helped him experience success that he could build upon. Have you ever felt really disappointed in yourself when you didn't fulfill a commitment you made to yourself or others? Nobody is perfect. It's natural to occasionally choose to do something else during the time you may have set aside to exercise, or to eat or drink foods you think are "bad." But if you then feel bad about yourself for messing up, what often happens next? Possibly you eat more or drink more. Or you feel terrible. Maybe you even call yourself names, like a fat failure.

The whole situation is a destructive cycle that we perpetuate through thoughts and beliefs about ourselves. It would be like purposively cutting our own rope while trying to climb a mountain. It's just a little counterproductive...okay...really counterproductive, to your goals and goal setting. If you're going to climb a mountain you want to ensure your ropes are strong and secure. If you're negatively judging yourself or your actions, you can guarantee that you are weakening your ropes, or in other words, your goals. You are going to set yourself up to be unsuccessful.

So let's talk about how to strengthen your resolve and increase your success. First off, we're human and therefore going to make mistakes or slip up, and that's okay. Again, we can be accountable for these moments, but don't need to be judgmental about them. Let's actually take a moment to define what I'm referring to with judgments.

For the purpose of this book, judgmentalism means defining or placing a value on an action, situation, behavior, etc., and deciding if it's right or wrong, good or bad, and so on. For example, while at a large fancy dinner, Jason sat at the honored guests table in front of a large crowd who were focused on those at the table. In this most uncomfortable situation, Jason was doing his best to mind his manners, but of course, being him, he accidentally hit the fork that was lying on his plate. It slid under some food and went flying towards the person on his right, splattering her with food. Red spaghetti sauce, noodles, and a few chunks of meatball splayed across her dress.

He was horrified. Immediately Jason began to define the situation, thinking of what a clumsy fool he was. The thoughts brought out his anxieties, and made him feel like garbage. His negative judgments didn't help him in any way, but only served to make the situation worse as he screeched his chair across the floor, bringing on more onlookers, and dabbing a napkin where he shouldn't be dabbing. Only later could he reframe his perspective of the situation. He chose to see it for what it was, an accident that resulted in someone getting food on them. If he could've looked at the actions from the viewpoint of a neutral bystander instead of judging them as bad or negative, he may have been able to think clearer and make better choices and acted appropriately instead of overreacting and feeling like a complete fool. Nobody else judged him as harshly as he judged himself. Nobody else thought the situation was as terrible as he made it out to be in his mind. They saw it as a human accident and laughed it off, thinking very little of it.

Let's look at the two examples earlier; what would be the negative judgments that they should remove? Right! Jason's good friend might want to remove the thought that she should've lost weight already and the gentlemen might want to remove the thought that he should be doing a lot more than what he could realistically do? Instead of focusing on negative judgments about what you should be and what you should be doing, be excited about who you are, what you can be, and what you are accomplishing. Those are all remarkable things, miracles in their own right. Look at the example in the graphic on the next page. More specifically, lets look at number three. In our society, tempting food is available everywhere. Let's say you see a fresh, warm doughnut and your thoughts get the best of you. You eat the donut, and then define your actions, judging them as bad. This makes it even harder to deal with the situation and achieve the outcome you want. The rope that you are using to climb the mountain begins to weaken.

Anything you can do to interrupt the cycle will make an impact; it will keep that rope strong. So to tackle this part of the cycle, you want to use a simple formula. Stop, remove judgment, take accountability (without judgment), refocus on the outcome, and decide on the path to get there.

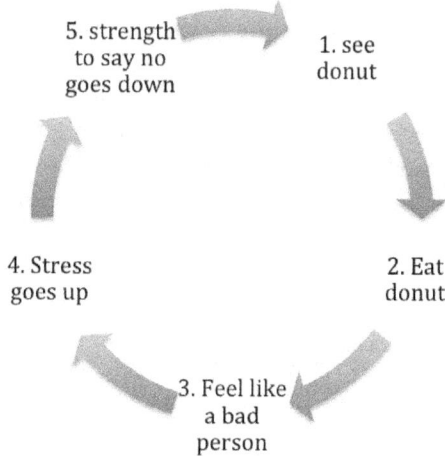

Stop! In order to stop, you often need to first see that you're thinking negatively about your actions or that you're judging yourself. When you notice having thoughts that your actions were bad or wrong, you need to literally stop and take a breath. Maybe even go sit down for a moment so you can take hold of your thoughts. We often overwhelm our minds by doing even more instead of just taking a breath. You might want to put a quote on the fridge that says, "Judgmentalism only makes the problem worse" to remind you to stop and ask what you are thinking about and remember to take a breath.

Remove the Judgment. Once you stop and possibly even sit down, the next step is to get rid of the judgment. Remind yourself that what you did wasn't bad, wrong, or the end of the world. It was just an action that you took. It doesn't need to be defined.

Do you have judgmental thoughts when the wind blows your fence down, or do you see what happened and then make preparations to fix it? Normally people just see what happened, possibly feel frustrated, and fix the problem. So, why don't we do that with ourselves? Instead of trying to define the action or give it meaning, accept what you have done and take steps to do something about it, that is, if you need to do something about it. Mistakes happen. They're absolutely human. There is no need to add judgment when you make a mistake.

Take Accountability. Accountability is holding yourself responsible for your thoughts and behaviors. Jason once worked with a client in counseling who arrived at the point where he was able to eliminate his judgmental thoughts, but he went a little too far and absolved himself of a key piece to success: accountability. Needless to say, he began to make choices that made life harder in the long run. He began to do whatever he wanted without looking at the outcomes of his actions.

Remember, your life is an accumulation of choices and circumstances. If you choose to smoke there will be outcomes such as cancer, premature aging, or other illnesses that follow. If you're mean to others, an outcome might be that no one wants to be near you. If you choose to eat poorly and not get enough physical activity, you will become out of shape and not as healthy as someone who eats well and exercises regularly. Obviously addiction and other mental/emotional problems may impinge on your ability to choose, making it more difficult to make wise choices. But no matter your circumstances, you can learn to make choices that move you to the outcomes that you are looking to accomplish.

Accountability is essential to help boost us into the life we want. It plays a crucial role in your success with Action Goals and outcomes. For example, not to long ago, Jason really wanted to get in shape and be healthier. It was a great desire of his, however, the choices he was making were leading him in the opposite direction. He led a very sedentary life. If what he wanted was to end up less healthy and fit, then he was doing a great job. On the other hand if he was going to be really serious about the outcome he wanted, he needed to be accountable for his actions. Knowing this, he reassessed his Action Goals, changed some of his eating habits, began working out, and held himself accountable for his choices.

So again, through our choices, we become what we are. Accountability helps us align those choices with the outcomes we want. Sometimes accountability can be hard to digest, but don't let that stop you from facing it. Everyone has a hard time looking at where they could do better. Nonetheless, growth only happens if you can do so. Look at yourself closely, and if you don't like what you find, take a breath and remind yourself that it's okay. After all, your Action Goals will help you get to the point where you really do live in alignment with your values.

There are many different ways to help keep ourselves accountable. We could keep charts that show what we are accomplishing, or we could involve others and let them know of our accomplishments. You can also keep a journal or use the Action Goal journal in this book. We always recommend that you share your goals and accomplishments with others.

Refocus Your Outcome. As mentioned in the last section, it's a good idea to take the time and ask yourself, "What do I want to get out of my life?" or "What do I want to accomplish with my health and weight loss?" You can write down the outcomes you want on the Action Goal chart provided.

It's hard to get somewhere if you don't know where that somewhere is. Do you want to lose five, ten, twenty, 100, or 200 pounds? Or maybe you want to be able to do an activity that you haven't done in a long time or possibly have never been able to do. These are all outcomes, and very important to have in your mind, or preferably, written down. They aren't to be confused with an Action Goal. Reminder, Action Goals are something you can do today while outcomes are products of our goals.

When setting an outcome, notice how it makes you feel. If you don't believe you will ever achieve the outcome, you will likely have little hope and feel deflated or you might want to give up. However, when you set an outcome and you continue to work on your Action Goals, it's only a matter of time before you will achieve your outcome. Keep in your mind that you CAN achieve the outcome—don't allow thoughts that your outcome is unattainable creep into your mind. Action Goals will work for you if you commit to them and refuse to give up.

Path To Get there. We have now arrived at the fun part. What will be your path to get there? Setting your Action Goals is just like charting the path you will take as you climb a mountain. You want to choose the easiest path that will get you to the top. Surprisingly, you don't have to choose the hard way. Please refer back to the chapter on Action Goals if you need to review how to set a successful plan. Below are different aspects to think about as you work on your Action Goals so you can be successful and disrupt the cycle so you can develop a new path.

Failing. Remember when we brought up that failing is a mythical word? Well it is, or at least it should be. Take it out of your vocabulary right now. This doesn't mean that you won't have setbacks or make mistakes, but setbacks and mistakes are not a failure. People who are most successful with weight loss are the ones who persevere through ups and downs. You always have another chance.

The moment we often define as a "failure" is actually a golden moment to help increase our chance of success. We are people of habit and we often make the same mistakes over and over. It's like continuously climbing the same bad part of a cliff where the rocks are too loose to get a good grip. If a rock climber notices that certain types of cliffs are unsafe to climb, he will learn to stay away from those areas. If we have a "failed" moment, then we have a perfect opportunity to stop and learn so we can do our best to make sure the situation doesn't happen again.

For example, Johnny wanted to lose 60 pounds. He set a goal to start working out with light weights. Both of his knees were bad so he didn't have many options. His specific goal was to lift weights every other evening for 30 minutes while watching TV. He had a great plan set up. However, when he came back the next week he was crushed. He didn't accomplish his goal.

"I completely failed," he explained to Jason. Thinking he knew what Jason was going to say next, he quickly added, "And I know it was a failure. I'm just a failure."

After discussing his feelings and thoughts, he and Jason worked on seeing "failed" moments as learning opportunities. Johnny identified what got in the way and what he could do differently to experience success. Since he identified he had a strong habit to just turn the TV on and forget about working out, he decided to keep the weights on the end table next to his remote so he remembered to start lifting when he turned the TV on.

The "failed" moment turned into a learning moment. He adjusted what he felt could make a difference and took action, which led to success. However, it took him having "failed" moments and looking at them as learning moments before he could come up with a more effective Action Goal. That's why those moments are such golden opportunities if utilized properly.

Our failures, after all, offer us a great chance to be successful next time. The story goes that Thomas Edison failed 1,000 times when trying to create the light bulb. To this, Edison supposedly said, "I have not failed 1,000 times. I have discovered 1,000 ways *not* to make a light bulb." When you look at your goals with the eyes of Edison, there are no failures, only chances to learn what to do differently next time.

So just remember that the moments you feel you have failed are actually crucial moments for you to learn and change the life patterns that have kept you from succeeding. Not only does a positive outlook help keep you motivated, it will also help you develop better Action Goals to be successful.

One step at a time. While writing his first book, there were many times that Jason basically gave up and put it to the side. He kept getting deflated because he wanted to finish it, yet kept focusing on how much he still had to do—all the chapters left to write, followed by editing the entire work. Because he was mostly focused on how far he had to go, he didn't get anywhere very fast. It took him almost ten years to write the book.

When he finally realized he needed to stop looking at everything that needed to be done and just focus on the piece of the book that he could write and work on that day, he found that he excelled. It's the same as the cliff climber. If she's focused on what she's doing in the moment, with awareness of her desired outcome, she has success. But when the climber changes her focus to everything around her and how far she still has to go, that's where she can get into trouble.

Sustained small steps daily bring about the big results we're looking for. When we apply this approach, we find that bigger things come. Whether it's getting a degree, getting a job, having a family, running a program, building a business, losing weight, or getting in shape, we achieve outcomes by the small daily steps that it takes to get there. Avoid the pitfall of looking at a huge project all together. Instead break down the steps and look at which one you need to start today.

Don't overwhelm yourself. There's more than one reason that taking small steps is important. Many times as a counselor, Jason would have parents walk through the door with small children in tow and explain that they'd had it with their child. Of course, he would have them explain the situation. One common example was that their child wouldn't clean their room. Parents would explain that they had taken all of the toys away and given every consequence they could think of and still the child wouldn't clean the room.

After listening to the situation, Jason would suggest the parents give the toys back because this step wasn't effective in getting the child to clean his room. Then he would suggest that the parents take the child into the room and let him know what reward he will get for cleaning it, and then ask the child to pick up a very specific toy or book and tell them where in the room it belonged. Jason would explain about being very specific because little children don't have the ability to do a large task without becoming instantly overwhelmed. They look at the entire mess and it gridlocks them. They would do what Jason had done with his first book, think only of how much they had to do and not about the little steps they could take. To relieve this, the children needed help breaking down different tasks. The next week, parents often came back with a success story, and often seemed surprised by the accomplishment, believing they had exhausted all options.

Now, even though as adults cleaning our bedroom isn't necessarily overwhelming, we can feel extremely overwhelmed with other things like losing weight or having to "completely" change our diet. And just like children, if we become overwhelmed it can often gridlock us and make it difficult to do anything. We want to avoid this!

To prevent or overcome this overwhelming feeling:

1. Focus on your Action Goals. Don't focus on the amount of weight you need to lose.
2. Make sure to set Action Goals that you can confidently say, "I believe with 90% certainty that I can accomplish this."
3. There are a lot of great ideas, but don't get sucked into the trap of setting too many goals. Don't set more than three Action Goals at a time. If they are bigger goals, you might want to keep it to one or two.

Don't keep temptation around. When Jason goes to the movie theatre, he always tells his wife that he would prefer to buy nothing—no treats or drinks. There is a simple purpose for this. When she buys popcorn, even if he doesn't plan on eating any, he finds himself mindlessly putting handfuls in his mouth. The same thing happens at home if he has a bag of chips out while watching a show or movie. Even worse, when he has soda pop in the house he drinks it instead of water.

You're probably nodding your head knowing exactly what Jason's talking about. Well, we're glad to say there is a simple solution to make eating healthier, easier. Are you ready? Don't buy it in the first place. Keep it out of the house. If it's not there, it's pretty hard to eat or drink it. When it's out of hand's reach then it won't end up in our hands. If your family members/spouse/loved ones are fighting with you about this, take time to sit down and explain how hard this makes it on you. Ask them if they could please support you in your goals so you can succeed. Let them know how important it is to you.

If you have a hard time at the store not buying the items, see if someone else would do the shopping which could help you reach your goals. You could also find someone to go with you and help keep you accountable for what you buy. If you don't have anyone to go for or with you, see if there's someone that you can call for support. Tell them what you will be buying and when you get back, let them know how well you did. Remember, having support can help you achieve success. Yes, we know we've said it already. But, it's that important.

One other way you can try to help keep yourself strong while at the store, which is discussed more in depth in a different chapter, is to shop the perimeter of the store and only the aisles with healthier food options. Don't go down the aisles that display junk foods that you know you'll be tempted to buy.

One client Jason was working with once told him he, "should be strong enough not to eat the junk food in the house." We have two things to say about this way of thinking. First, it has a judgment: "Should." Second, there's no reason to make your goals harder by keeping foods around that are very hard to resist. We can all be strong for only so long before we give into temptations. Change is hard enough, there's no reason to make it harder. Make your Action Goals as easy as possible.

Positive vs. Negative. Choose a Positive Perspective. One sunny day while Jason sat in his home office writing, his three-year-old daughter approached him. Her small hands were cupped together with something inside that she had picked up while shopping with her mom. Without taking her eyes off her hidden prize, she just stood there smiling, proud of whatever it was.

"What do you have there?" Jason inquired.

"It's beautiful," she spoke softly, still not looking away.

"But what is it?" Jason persisted.

"It's my beautiful rock."

"Oh, can I see your beautiful rock?"

"It's beautiful," she repeated.

Finally, with her big smile she slowly opened her hands. Jason's expectations were high. Was it some kind of colorful or translucent rock? Or maybe even crystal-like? Nope—none of the above. It was a dirty plain brown rock. There wasn't one thing about it that Jason would have classified as beautiful.

"It's beautiful, right Dad?"

"Definitely!" Jason said with a smile.

Of course Jason didn't think the rock was beautiful, however, his daughter was teaching him a valuable lesson. She was showing him how to see beauty where most people don't. It all had to do with her perspective.

Perspective is an extremely important part of success. If Jason's daughter didn't think the rock was beautiful, she never would've picked it up. The rock would've stayed in the parking lot to be stepped on by customers at the store. The same is true with your goals and the life around you. If you aren't seeing the positive you often don't take action. If you look at the negative, this creates stress and makes it harder to achieve what we want. Thinking and acting positively moves you forward, it's proactive vs. negative thinking and talking, which takes us away and prohibits.

We see what we focus on. If we focus on the dirt and negativity in life then that's what we'll see. If we give attention to the beautiful and positive aspects of life then that's what we'll experience. In fact, life is what we make it.

Jason never realized how satisfaction in life is a direct consequence of perspective until he was living in the Kiribati Islands on the island of Tarawa. The locals lived in small huts that were off the ground and had no walls. They had very little in material terms, and yet they were some of the happiest people he ever met. They were content and grateful for what they had instead of being unhappy and negative about what they didn't. They took time to find value and beauty instead of noticing flaws. They saw positive in the negative and accepted life for what it was. Of course not every native islander looked at life with this perspective, but most did.

Here are a few tricks to help you stay positive as you pursue your goals.

1.   When you feel yourself being negative, stop and take a breath. Think about what is causing you to feel negative. Analyze the thought. Is it unrealistic? Try to take time to think about what the realistic thought is, or what a positive perspective can be and change your negative thought.

2.   If the first method doesn't work, then try doing something you love. Work in the garden, read a good book, take a walk, go fishing, call a good friend, or whatever it is that makes you feel good. Take time to relax and allow yourself to see the situation in a more helpful light.

Another area that can cause a lot of negative thinking is when we take things personally. This may not directly impact your goals and success, but may indirectly sabotage your efforts if these moments put you into a negative mindset, which can disrupt your goals.

For example Judy was extremely upset about hurtful things her teenage daughter said, such as, "I hate you mom," and "You're the worst mom ever. I can't wait to get away from you." Judy internalized these statements and it brought her down, causing her to go through the drive-thru and order super-sized meals.

Internalizing those things her daughter said would hurt any parent. Judy wasn't a bad mom. Sure, she had areas where she could improve her parenting to get better outcomes with her daughter, but nobody does things perfectly and the fact that she could improve didn't make her a bad mom. She loved her daughter and was trying her best. Remember, when we look at the things we need to change, we need to take out the judgment. If Judy had been the worst mom on the face of the Earth, that would've been a different story, but truly she wasn't.

Jason helped Judy look at what her daughter was probably feeling when she made those statements. Judy began to empathize with her daughter's feelings when she was grounded or the car was taken away. It's never fun to have a consequence, but that doesn't mean her daughter didn't need a consequence. Judy's daughter didn't truly hate Judy. Rather, her daughter was simply upset and reacting to the consequence. Judy saw that the statements didn't need to be internalized or taken personally. In fact, they weren't even about her. They were statements made from her daughter's anger.

When you feel yourself taking things personally, take a minute to stop and do at least two things.

1. Remember that it's not about you. It's about the other person's perspective and let them own that. This doesn't mean you should start arguing with them and not listen to their perspective. It just means you don't have to internalize it. You can still take time to try to appreciate and understand why they would be feeling the way they're feeling.
2. If there is some truth to what they are saying (for example, maybe you did something that was your fault), then take steps to apologize or determine how you might be able to make the situation better. But be careful not to judge yourself in these situations. Don't start defining yourself as a bad person. Just take accountability, change your behavior if necessary, and apologize.

Take a Time Out. Often times we're swamped in life, going from one thing, to another, to another. We neglect to take time to ponder what we're doing or what we'd like to do or be.

It may be hard to justify taking time to analyze your life. Laura told Jason it was hard for her to take a time out because all she could think of was everything she wasn't getting done. She didn't value time to let her mind take a break and collect itself.

While working on your goals, we hope you recognize how valuable it is to take time to reflect on your progress and ask yourself if you need to adjust your Action Goals. In fact, right now, pick a day and time each week when you can ponder your goals, maybe Saturday morning or Sunday night or Tuesday afternoon. Set aside this time to think about what exactly you were able to accomplish during the week. Ponder questions like:

Did I accomplish the goals? And if you did, enjoy the feeling of success for a moment.

Were they a struggle to accomplish?
Or were they too easy?
Do I need to make modifications?
If you weren't able to accomplish your goals, what did you learn and what will you do next time to be more successful?

Now it's your turn. At the back of this book, on page 55, your Action Goal Journal begins. The first page is for your starting goal. The following pages are separated for you to review your goal each week. There are extra "New Goal" sheets in case you feel you are ready to set new goals, however, don't feel obligated to add more if you aren't ready.

CHAPTER THREE

You Can Have It All

You can eat anything and still lose weight—*anything!* From pizza to french fries to pasta to cheesecake, no foods are off limits. This concept isn't new, but a lot of people have a really hard time believing it.

It's not your fault if you have occasionally bought into the belief that you had to ban certain foods in order to lose weight. Even though the Academy of Nutrition and Dietetics, the world's largest organization of food and nutrition professionals, preaches moderation, pop culture still embraces an all-or-nothing diet approach.

Think of the popular weight loss shows and books. They often recommend extreme approaches, more radical than anyone living a real life can realistically follow. Most of us aren't going to scale Mount Everest. Likewise, most of us aren't going to see success on the next fad diet and become the diet's spokesperson either.

Still, people want immediate results. They want to believe in the power of something outside of themselves to fix their weight problem. Who can blame them? We are used to having everything instantly, from email, to music, to microwave meals. Have you ever forbidden your favorite food? If so, how long were you able to give it up? You may have denied yourself for a period of days, weeks, or even months, but eventually a craving for the food you love will began to build. Did you end up giving in and overdoing it? If so, don't take this as a personal failing. Most people who cut out their favorite foods ultimately eat more in the long run, sabotaging their weight loss efforts.

If you think you can't have a certain food, there's probably going to come a point where you really, *really* want it. At this perilous point, you might go off your diet and eat all the foods that you have denied yourself.

So, if you have to ban a food, ban only foods you don't like.

Holly struggled for years with overeating, and it was largely because of this good vs. bad mentality. She was either on her eating plan or completely, absolutely off her eating plan. When she was on, her diet was extremely restrictive. She ate perfectly—in her mind at least. Her perfect diet consisted only of healthy foods like whole grain cereals, skim milk, dried beans, and lots of fruit and vegetables.

Sadly, nobody's perfect, and expecting herself to eat perfectly was a set-up for failure. Just when she thought she was getting close to reaching the top of the mountain, she'd get so sick and tired of depriving herself that she'd give in and go hog-wild, eating anything and everything fattening and delicious— especially if it included chocolate. After free falling until she hit rock bottom, she'd start all over again, convincing herself that this time she wouldn't lose traction. This time she'd keep a firm grip on her strict diet and make it to the top. This time would be different.

Of course, it never was. Einstein said the definition of insanity is doing the same thing over and over again and expecting different results. Holly did this for years. Sometimes, she'd plan to stay on her eating plan, but then she'd get talked out of it, like when she succumbed to peer pressure and had a piece of cake at a friend's birthday. Then she'd figure she totally blew it with one piece of cake, so she may as well go buy a whole cake and eat it all by herself! Back to the ground she would fall.

Holly didn't have success with weight loss until she finally, genuinely believed that no foods were bad. In other words, she did something *different*. She stopped banning the food she loved.

You really don't have to deprive yourself to lose weight. In fact, most people gain back the weight they lose on strict eating plans, and often gain even more. Nevertheless, people continue to spend huge amounts of money on weight loss products such as diet food and supplements. These products may work for the short-run, but in the long run, the only thing that ends up thinner is their bank account.

If you live for hamburgers, then make sure to include hamburgers in your Action Goals. You might make it a goal to have one hamburger every week.

Kelly was eating two packs of Oreos a week (that's 102 cookies total) and solemnly swore that they were her number one pleasure in life. When we first met, Kelly wanted to lose weight badly for a couple of reasons. First, she was single and hoping to get a boyfriend. Second, she thought weight loss would help to increase her confidence.

The problem was that Kelly did not want (nor was she ready) to cut Oreos completely from her diet. With help she began to see this wasn't really a problem. She could still have Oreos. Together, we decided that she would simply cut back to 84 Oreos a week (seven a day).

This may seem like a trivial step, but it wasn't at all. Previously, she had been eating, on average, 14 Oreos a day! Just by this small change, she wiped out 490 calories a day. She decided to replace the seven Oreos she eliminated with two apples every day. Her two apples amounted to 140 calories. When you do the math, she cut out 490 calories of Oreos daily and added in 140 calories of apples, so she ended up eating 350 fewer calories every day just by eating apples in place of some of her Oreos.

Kelly's results from this one small change were amazing. She lost between one-half to one pound every week for the first three months that we worked together. After three months of doing nothing but this one small change, she had lost about eight pounds. Spurred on by her results, she decided that she wanted to begin walking for twenty minutes every day and that she only wanted to eat four Oreos a day. Over the next three months, she lost around 18 more pounds. Her original outcome goal was to lose 25 pounds, and she succeeded easily in six months by taking small steps.

Now the really good news. She found walking to be even more pleasurable than eating Oreos. She ranked walking above the Oreos because she felt so good about herself after a walk. But here's the best news of all. Though she'll never consider herself a social butterfly, Kelly's weight loss did make her feel better about herself, and in turn, she got together with her friends more often. At one gathering, she was introduced to a man who—can you guess? ... has become her husband! To this day, she has maintained her weight loss.

Remember, no foods are off limits. If this sounds too good to be true, know that it's really not. You *can* have your cake and eat it too—and get thinner to boot!

CHAPTER FOUR

Enjoy Every Bite

Food is meant to be eaten with gusto, to be fully savored and enjoyed. It is one of the great gifts that we get to experience as human beings. Sadly, many people have come to believe that they can't enjoy their food and also stay thin and healthy, too. They think that food shouldn't taste too good or they won't be able to stop eating. They think that everything that tastes good will make them fat.

Actually, it's not the food, but how we are thinking about the food, that leads us to struggle with food and weight. The next time you eat, allow yourself to be fully present and experience the food. Eat it with attention, focus, and most importantly, without a trace of guilt. This way of eating takes practice, but over time if you commit to noticing your judgments about eating, you can teach yourself to eat with freedom.

Many people eat most of their meals while doing something else, and thus only devote a portion of their attention to their food. If you answer yes to any of the following questions, it may be that you aren't giving yourself the opportunity to *really* relish your food.

- Do you eat in your car while driving?
- Do you eat while reading or watching TV?
- Do you eat at your desk while working?
- Do you sneak food so others won't see you and it eat in a rush?
- Do you eat while you're cleaning the house or doing dishes?
- Do you eat standing up?

A mountain climber must maintain complete focus on the task at hand. They can't climb a mountain and check out the latest online news at the same time or they may end up plunging to their death. Luckily, if you lose your focus while eating it's probably not going to kill you, but it will likely make it harder to lose weight.

Eat with all of your senses. When you see a substantial meal laid out on the table before you, it gives your brain the message that you will be satisfied when you are finished eating. If your plate of food is colorful and attractive, then you subconsciously believe that you are treating yourself to something nice. If you believe you are eating a satisfying amount of food, then you will not feel as much need to overeat.

If you eat from a bag or a jar, your eyes can't see how much you are eating. It may sound silly, but you won't be satisfying your eyes. This will quite possibly lead to eating more food than you really need.

When you eat, EAT, and do nothing else. If you eat while engaged in another activity, such as watching television or checking email, much of your brain is focused on what you are doing or observing and NOT on what you are eating. Sure, the food probably still tastes good, but it isn't as satisfying as it could be if you were totally focused on the flavor, smell, texture, and even the sound it makes. If you eat when you are not fully paying attention to the food and process of eating, then your senses are only half-engaged. As a result, you will probably need more to feel satisfied. Eating while doing something else usually results in overeating.

Make a production out of eating. This doesn't mean that preparing food has to take all kinds of time. You don't have to cook yourself a gourmet meal (unless you want to). Just begin to appreciate the sensuality of food before you put it in your mouth. If you do cook, take time to notice the shapes, colors, and texture of various foods. If your meal is from a can or box, then present it nicely on the plate and sit down at the table to eat it.

S-l-o-w down while you eat. Before you put anything in your mouth, tell yourself you are going to take time to savor it. Consider eating with your non-dominant hand to help ensure a more leisurely pace. Just watch out for spills!

Chew your food well. The more you take your time with food, the less need you will have to overeat.

Let your body be the boss. Strict diets often take the control of eating away from the body and give it to the mind. The diet decides when and what you can eat. You ignore your body's cues for the sake of rules you believe you must follow.

Sam was a dream client. As a brand new dietitian, Holly was thrilled that he listened to all of her suggestions and agreed with everything she had to say. She told him to eat no more than 2,000 calories per day and to get at least 30 minutes of exercise five days a week. Wanting to please her and lose weight fast, he decided to eat only 1,000 calories per day and workout for one hour.

Holly and Sam talked weekly, and he consistently lost 5 to 6 pounds a week. In no time (actually about two months) he lost fifty pounds and became quite thin. Both of them were happy with the results and terminated the sessions.

Three months later, Sam called Holly and said he was doing terribly. He had gained all the weight back, plus ten pounds. Inexperienced and unaware of how common it is for dieters to regain their lost weight, Holly was shocked and disheartened to hear that Sam had put sixty pounds back on. Sam then told Holly the truth. He had lost the weight by nearly starving himself. He said he had felt hungry all the time while he was dieting, and after he lost the weight he figured he could finally eat again.

At that point in Holly's career, she wasn't aware of how important it was to honor true hunger. Rather than telling Sam to impose an arbitrary calorie goal, she could have helped him listen to his body's cues and let his body decide how much he needed to eat. Now, remember, calories do count! You need to reduce your total calorie intake in order to lose weight. But if you eat too few calories and starve your body, you may end up slowing down your metabolism and weighing even more in the long run. Sam cut calories back to the point that he was miserable, and this only resulted in a huge drive to overeat when he went off the strict diet.

Can you remember a time when food and eating were not an issue in your life? Was there a time when you could eat whatever you wanted and you felt good about your body?

If so, why did you eat during this time of ease?

Most likely you ate because your body was truly hungry. You can return to this time. You can reclaim a healthy, joyous relationship with food. The key to doing so is to begin to trust your body when it tells you *when to eat* and *when to stop* eating.

The body wants to survive and thrive. It's not going to give the critical function of eating to the mind without a fight. If you decide not to eat when your body is hungry, your body will likely drive you to overeat later. If you decide to eat celery when your body really needs energy from carbohydrates, the body will continue to let you know it's lacking the critical nutrients that it needs. It will ramp up appetite hormones in the hopes that you feed it something with carbohydrates. Give control back to your body, where it belongs, and your body will be far less likely to drive you to overeat.

After you finish eating, you should feel better than you felt before you began eating. Many people who overeat feel worse after they finish eating than before they began eating. If you can stop eating when your hunger is gone, but before you are full or stuffed, then you have eaten just the right amount for optimal energy. Of course, learning to stop eating when you are satisfied can be very difficult. It takes practice.

You can't scale a mountain without plenty of guidance and practice. Likewise, you need guidance and practice to change your eating habits. The sections below offer valuable techniques to help you learn to eat just enough.

Welcome your cravings. Stop to think before you eat, checking in with yourself for a second or two to notice whether you are truly physically hungry. If you are, then it's time to eat. At this point, ask yourself what you feel like eating. Do you want something warm or cold? Crunchy or smooth? Comforting or exotic? Savory, sweet, salty, or spicy? Think about what type of food would satisfy you the most.

Also, think about how the food will affect your body. Will it give your body the nutrition it needs? Will it make you feel good after you eat it? Often, if you think about what the food actually does in your body, you'll find you'd rather choose something healthy and high quality. Ask: (1) Is this food a good quality fuel. (2) What will my cells do with the food? (3) Will this food provide the nutrients my body needs to repair and restore my tissues and help me stay young?

You need brightly colored fruits and vegetables for their anti-cancer effects. You need whole grains and dried beans for the added fiber that helps protect against disease. You need lean protein to restore your body's tissues while keeping your heart healthy.

As you gain a heightened awareness of the profound impact nutritious food has on your health, then eating healthy becomes a treat in itself. It feels really good to treat your body—unarguably your most valuable possession—right.

Of course, sometimes you may find that you really want something just for the pleasure it offers. It's okay to eat less healthy food about 20 percent of the time if the other 80 percent of the time you are loading your body up with foods high in vitamins and minerals. In fact, it's better to satisfy a strong craving than to let it intensify until you give in and gorge.

When you make a conscious decision that what you are eating is something you really want, then you'll find it much easier to stop with a smaller amount of food. Sometimes people deliberately ignore their cravings. They may tell themselves they have what they really want. And so they end up eating all kinds of other foods in attempt to satisfy their desires. But all the other—often-healthier—foods don't hit the spot, and in the end they just give in eat what they want after consuming hundreds of calories of healthy food first. They'd be much better off satisfying their craving first versus eating excessively in attempt to satisfy their craving with foods that can't satisfy. Just because a food is healthy, doesn't mean it won't go straight to your thighs or waistline if you eat too much.

Let go of tomorrow's diet. Have you ever eaten in a last chance sort of way? This happens when you tell yourself something like, "I already blew it by eating one cookie, so I may as well eat the whole bag. I'll never eat cookies again after this. Tomorrow I'll start my diet. *Stick to salads, I will!"* Saying that last sentence in Yoda-speak may even temporarily convince you that you'll have the power of the force to follow through.

And the next day, or few days, or even few weeks, you might stick to a strict plan. But after a while, you'll start to get tired of depriving yourself. You may start to notice fear arising along with the following types of thoughts:
- "How long will I have to be deprived?"

- "This is hard."
- "I'm tired of being so disciplined."
- "What if I can't stick to my perfect eating plan? Then I'll be in trouble."

Were you ever told there was something you couldn't do and just being told this made you really want to do it? That's exactly what a strict diet does.

At some point in their diet, most people decide that it is too hard and restrictive. They decide to go off their diet. Sometimes, they go off their diet in secretive ways. They sneak food when no one else can see them, or even deceive themselves by refusing to admit that they really ate *that* much.

Sandra was considerably overweight and she believed that if she ate anything fattening in front of others, they would think poorly of her. Her mom and dad were always watching and telling her what she should or shouldn't eat. Her well-meaning friends did the same, pointing out healthier foods and asking her how her diet was going. Sandra wanted others to know that she really was trying to lose weight so whenever she went to a family meal or a dinner party with friends, she only ate very small amounts of super healthy food. But inside, she resented others for making her feel as though she had to be good all of the time.

Of course, Sandra was ultimately in charge of what she did or did not put into her mouth, and her family and friends couldn't really stop her from eating all of the good food that they were enjoying right in front of her. However, Sandra had a deep-seated fear that she would not be acceptable if she ate high-calorie food given her current weight. So, she always showed the world her best eating habits, while inside she seethed and waited for her chance to indulge.

After shared meals with family and friends, Sandra would often offer to clean up while her host relaxed, and in the kitchen alone, she would sneak bites of the lasagna or cheesecake or whatever she could find. She would stuff the food in her mouth and swallow it whole in an attempt to go undiscovered. Or she would swing by fast food after her gatherings and order a supersized meal. She looked forward to the opportunity to finally satisfy her desires, but also felt guilty for her behavior. While she ate, she promised herself that *tomorrow* her diet would start for good. After she finished eating, Sandra always felt guilty and like a fraud. She hated herself for her actions. But she didn't know how to break the cycle. She'd be "good" the next day or few days only to lose control once again.

Through counseling, Sandra learned to feel comfortable enough to eat what she wanted in front of anyone. She deserved to enjoy her food regardless of her weight. Gradually, she came to believe that she was just as worthy as anyone else of eating and enjoying good food. When she gave herself permission to have it openly, she found that she didn't need as much to satisfy her. She realized it was never satisfying or enjoyable to eat in a frenzied, secretive sort of way that allowed her no chance to take her time and savor her meal.

Unfortunately, eating secretly and guiltily means that while indulging in your favorite treats, you're also feeling bad. You're aware that you are really blowing it. You're letting yourself down. You're acting in a self-destructive way, sabotaging your ultimate goal to achieve a healthier body and state of mind. And after you finish eating, you feel even worse. You're full of remorse and self-disgust. Naturally, you promise yourself that you'll get back on the restrictive eating plan, which then sets you up for another slip-up. Can you see how it becomes a vicious cycle?

If you find yourself in a cycle of dieting followed by overeating, please know that beating yourself up about it won't change it. Being hard on yourself only creates more pain, and the last thing you deserve is more pain about your eating habits and weight. Instead, promise yourself that diets and restriction are in your past. Because when you truly believe food will always be there for you, food loses its power—it's no longer so darn tempting.

When you know that you can eat whenever you really want or need food in front of anybody (YES! You are beautiful, wonderful, and valuable enough to eat whatever you like and it's everybody else's problem if they don't like it), then your anxiety about food and eating may fall away. You know, letting other people determine what you can and can't eat really does keep you from making healthy choices. Part of losing weight for good means trying hard not to care what other people think and honoring your needs in each moment. When you know that you can have food, of course you'll still want it—we all need it—but not so powerfully and painfully. And you'll need less to satisfy you. If, while eating you're favorite food, you tell yourself that the diet starts tomorrow and this is your last chance to enjoy the food, you will undoubtedly want to eat as much as you can.

Try not to think too far into the future when it comes to making changes to your diet. Instead, focus your attention on each day, or better yet, each moment. Think, "What can I do today to achieve my Action Goal?" If you can stay on track just for today without worrying about tomorrow, you'll be surprised how far you can go.

If you start to worry about tomorrow, you may find that you develop a lot of anxiety over your ability to stick with positive changes. It all might become overwhelming. Likewise, if you slipped up yesterday and are feeling like a failure, you might start to think that you can't achieve your goals. At these points, you are at BIG risk for giving up—for falling halfway down the face of the cliff.

So forget yesterday, forget tomorrow, and just do your best TODAY! Make tiny little changes that allow you to enjoy life and food as you lose weight. One little, calculated step up the mountain at a time will get you to the top.

Keep healthy food on hand. It's a good idea to stock your home with lots of healthy food that you enjoy, but that you aren't necessarily tempted to eat in excess. Include foods like whole grains, lean protein, fruits, vegetables, raw nuts, and legumes. If necessary, buy food that is quick and easy to prepare so when you are hungry you will have something readily available.

You might also keep a little stash of your favorite junk. Besides having healthy foods on hand, consider also having some treats (food that's not necessarily healthy, but that you really enjoy). At the same time, limit the amount of high calorie food you purchase. Stick to one or two junk foods in your home at one time, and keep them out of sight. It's human nature to be tempted by foods high in sugar, fat, and salt, especially if they are staring us in the face.

If a box of frosted cupcakes is sitting in plain view on the counter, it's likely you will be tempted to indulge. In fact, it takes a lot of effort not to indulge because humans are programmed to want to eat high-calorie food when it's available. This is a survival mechanism from the Stone Ages, when people needed to eat a lot of calories in order to store fat and survive times of famine. Now, we no longer have times of famine, but we still all like to eat.

If you find that you overeat when you have high-calorie sweet or fattening foods around, then plan to only eat them at a restaurant, or purchase only single-serving sizes. Also start to believe that at some point it may be possible to keep these foods in your house without overeating them. If you tell yourself you are someone who has no self-control, you will be someone with no self-control. On the other hand, if you tell yourself you are someone with a lot of self-control (or even that you are learning self-control), over time you'll probably be able to eat tempting foods in moderation. You will be able to have a normal portion and then walk away.

Redefine yourself as someone in control. Don't let negative thoughts about yourself dictate your eating behavior. You can set yourself up for successful weight loss by making it easy to eat healthy foods and limiting treats, while at the same time telling yourself that you can eat whatever you really want. Just because you have overeaten in the past doesn't mean you are not free to choose differently now.

Breathe out a sigh of relief. The food fight can be over for good.

Know your deepest hungers. Often people eat to satisfy a hunger that has nothing to do with the need for food. Maybe it's a hunger for rest, or companionship, or fun, or new challenges. Because they don't know how, or think they can't, satisfy their true hungers, they put something in their mouth, hoping food will at least soothe them and make them forget that their life is lacking in other ways. But no amount of food can satisfy an emotional, mental, or even physical need (like the need for touch or intimacy).

Do you know the difference between physical hunger and emotional or mouth hunger? Physical hunger is true hunger. When you are physically hungry, your body is letting you know that it needs fuel and it's time to eat. When you are not physically hungry, you do not need to eat. Everybody eats for reasons that have nothing to do with true physical hunger sometimes. It's okay to eat just because you feel like it. *Occasionally*. However, some people eat for reasons other than true physical hunger *most* of the time. When you eat for psychological reasons most of the time, it can be hard to control your weight and can lead to a cycle of overeating and subsequently feeling bad about yourself.

Can you tell when you are truly physically hungry? Physical hunger is felt by a sense of emptiness in the stomach, and only occurs a few to several hours after a meal. When you are just starting to get physically hungry, you will feel a bit of emptiness in your stomach or a minor gnawing feeling. Your stomach may growl lightly. The longer you wait to eat, the hungrier you will get. The gnawing feeling intensifies, and your stomach may growl loudly. In other words, physical hunger builds gradually over time.

If you allow yourself to become overly hungry, you will likely start to feel signs of hunger elsewhere in your body. You might feel light-headed or experience a headache. You may become tired and crabby. Eventually, you might get to a point where you want to eat everything in sight.

If you find yourself in this place of extreme hunger, try to cultivate calmness by deep breathing or by focusing on relaxing your body before you start to eat. If you are in a frantic emotional state when you eat, you're eating will be frantic. It's critical to begin eating only when you are feeling at peace. This way, you will be much less likely to eat in an out-of-control manner.

To avoid the agitation that can result from extreme hunger, eat when you feel slight to moderate physical hunger and stop when you are satisfied, but not overly full. If you wait until you are starving, chances are good that you will eat too much. Likewise, if you eat until you are stuffed, you'll probably ingest more calories than your body needs and your body may end up storing some (or many) of these calories as fat.

In contrast to eating for physical hunger, many people eat for psychological reasons. There are so many reasons people eat that have nothing to do with hunger! Often when people eat for reasons other than physical hunger, they feel guilty or angry with themselves afterward. **Clients have often said, "I eat because I feel bad, and then I feel even worse for eating so much, so I eat some more."**

Here are ten reasons people eat besides physical hunger. You need to know these reasons because awareness of behavior and insight into our mind is the first step required to changing for good. See if any of these apply to you:

1. **To ease or avoid physical pain.** Have you suffered a physical injury and eased it with a treat? Beginning in childhood, many people learn to ease physical pain with an ice cream cone or a sweet. For example, you hurt yourself or had to get your tonsils out, and were rewarded with something good to eat.

2. **To ease or avoid emotional pain.** Eating can help you cope with stress, depression, loneliness, and a whole host of negative emotions. While you're eating, you temporarily feel better. Unfortunately, just like any addiction, after you finish eating you usually feel worse. You may feel so bad about eating that you continue eating because you feel guilty for eating. This creates a vicious cycle.

3. **To alleviate boredom or apathy.** When you feel aimless and don't know what to do with yourself, food can fill up your time. It can even make you too tired to do anything, thus giving you an excuse to continue feeling bored or apathetic.

4. **To provide a reward for hard work.** Food is frequently used as a reward. You might think:
   - "I had a stressful day, so I deserve a gourmet meal out."
   - "I'm studying hard for this test. I've earned some pizza."
   - "I made it through that grueling workout, and now I can have a milkshake."

5. **To celebrate.** From birthdays to holidays to graduations, food is an inherent part of celebration. In our society, a party without good food just wouldn't be the same.

6. **To follow an eating plan or diet.** If you are on a diet plan, it may tell you when it's time for breakfast, lunch, or dinner. You are following the plan and not your internal hunger cues. If the diet only allows certain foods, then you are not listening to your desires.

7. **To increase energy or alertness.** When you are tired, food can provide a temporary energy boost. Your body really needs sleep, but you use food to keep going instead. The act of chewing or sucking can keep you awake and alert. You know this first hand if you've ever bought snacks to keep from nodding off during a long drive.

8. **To satisfy a craving.** Food is a very sensual experience. It can look beautiful, smell wonderful, taste delicious, feel great in your mouth (creamy, crunchy, smooth, soft, chewy), and can even sound scrumptious. Think of the successful advertising for Rice Krispies: snap, crackle, pop! Because it appeals to all of our senses, it can be very hard to resist.

9. **To ward off potential threats.** Some people eat because their weight, either consciously or subconsciously, keeps them safe. People who have been sexually abused or assaulted often gain weight so that they appear less attractive and thus less likely to be a sexual target in the future.

10. **To keep unwelcome behaviors in check.** This is similar to eating to avoid emotional pain, only rather than using food to soothe your internal emotions you are using food to control your external behavior. You might be angry but you don't want to unleash your anger on another person. So you stuff your anger with a brownie. Or you might be sad but you don't want others to see you crying, so you dry your tears with a sandwich.

If you are eating mostly for psychological reasons, it is critical that you begin to be *kind* to yourself. After overeating, most people berate themselves. They call themselves nasty names or feel totally defeated by their lack of willpower. If you judge yourself harshly or become angry with yourself after overeating, then it will be very hard to change your behavior for good.

It's better to just be curious and try to figure out what led you to overeat. You must know the cause before you can address your behavior. Allow all of your thoughts and emotions to surface. Rather than completely identifying with your thoughts and letting them take you over, just watch your mind. Notice your feelings. Become aware of why you ate. As mentioned above, *awareness is the first step to change.*

When Holly first met Erin (one of Holly's clients), Erin said that she didn't eat for any hidden reasons. "I just like food and enjoy eating too much." Erin had three young children and was a stay-at-home mom. She said she had a good marriage and a happy life. She was very involved in her kid's activities. Over time Erin revealed that she also suffered from fibromyalgia and lived with lots of pain in her joints. Nonetheless, she had to be active and on the go shuttling her children back and forth from school to their activities.

Over time Erin identified eating habits that were keeping her from losing weight. One habit was eating her children's leftovers. Erin knew not to make her kids clean their plates if they were no longer hungry, but she admitted that she often ate what they left: a few bites of macaroni and cheese, a quarter of a peanut-butter and jelly, and a swallow of chocolate milk. She hated wasting food.

Aha. Here was one reason she was eating other than for physical hunger or simple enjoyment.

Erin eating leftovers when she wasn't hungry would result in her body storing the extra calories as fat. So although she was minimizing waste in the garbage, she was adding to her own waist. She needed to decide which was more preferable, food waste or fat on her waist.

When considering it this way, Erin readily admitted that she'd rather throw food out than put it in her body where it would be stored as fat. We talked about how, in the long run, adding to her waist would be more costly in terms of health and emotional consequences (how she felt about herself). Erin then made the commitment to either put leftovers away for her children to eat later, or throw them away. She would no longer take on the role of personal cleanup crew and trash compactor.

Erin's only me-time during the day was naptime. With her oldest off at school and her two younger children snoozing, Erin relished this time. She'd grab a magazine and a big bowl of ice cream or cookies and enjoy herself. No doubt, Erin deserved downtime. However, rather than head straight to the magazine with treats in hand, she would sit down on the couch, take some deep breaths, and notice her thoughts and feelings for a few minutes, assuring her that after this step, she could indulge in reading and eating.

When Erin noted her feelings, she discovered that she was in significant physical pain. She was tired and achy and just wanted an escape. She realized treats helped distract her. They were a temporary reprieve from her aching body. We explored what else might help her feel better. She thought about it for a few days and decided a foot bath massager with sea salt and essential oil scrub would be really nice. From that point on, she used the foot bath massage during naptime with her magazine. She found she enjoyed it as much as the sweets. Cutting out her afternoon treats helped her finally lose the weight.

When you're not hungry, yet you find yourself at the refrigerator door, this is the perfect situation to learn about what it is you truly need. It's a chance to find the perfect foothold on the face of the cliff. It's a chance to grow into somebody who will reach the top of your life. Before you take a bite of food, sit with your desire. Embrace your craving. Where is it coming from within you? Is food acting as your friend? Is it soothing your stress? Are you overly tired? Do you lack direction or passion in your life? Has food become your main source of pleasure? What sense of lack are you trying to fill with food?

Once you know why you are eating, you can make a plan to address whatever area is deficient or needs attention in your life. If it's friends you need, how can you make some? Maybe buy a book on becoming a friend, or join an organization where you can meet people, or volunteer. One thing is certain, you won't make friends sitting at home eating.

If you're overstressed, how can you bring more peace to your days? Would it help to take a meditation class? Or yoga? Do you need time in the morning to pray? Maybe you have overcommitted yourself and need to cut back on daily duties. In this day and age there are so many ordinary humans expecting themselves to be superheroes.

There are many reasons why your life might be out of balance, and whenever life lacks balance, food becomes more attractive. It's critical that you work on underlying issues that are driving you to overeat. Seek out whatever help, information, and support you need. You can even call Holly or Jason for private therapy sessions to accelerate your success.

Find a New Drug of Choice. Food is not meant to be our main source of satisfaction in life. Yet for many people, it has become just that. In today's environment, high calorie, intensely flavorful food is available practically everywhere we look. It is readily accessible in places like convenient stores, restaurants, and vending machines, and it's easy to consume. Tasty food provides an easy way to make it through our fast-paced, sometimes empty lives. If you feel bored or down or stressed, a velvety chocolate bar or a bag of salty chips is a great distraction.

Food that is highly processed and contains artificial flavors and lots of sugar, salt, or fat makes us want it more and more. When we eat foods like pizza, chocolate, potato chips, or ice cream, they cause a release of certain chemicals in our body, primarily dopamine and serotonin, that bring us pleasure and drive us to eat. They work on us like a drug. So not only is the taste and texture of high calorie foods pleasurable, but they also enhance our appetite and mood *temporarily*. Consequently, many people end up overeating these types of food. Or they eat when they are not hungry for the brief little boost.

For many people, eating becomes their very favorite activity. It is a somewhat acceptable drug of choice.

If you eat highly processed food much of the time, you may find that more natural, healthy food tastes bland. But the good news is that our taste buds adapt to whatever we get used to eating. If you gradually choose less processed, healthier food without added sugar, salt, and fat, your taste buds will adapt to more natural food over time, and you will actually start to prefer healthy food.

Additionally, if you eat when you are hungry, your taste buds are more sensitive and food tastes better. You may have heard that hunger is the best seasoning. This has been proven. Food doesn't taste as good when we are full.

Start to limit your access to fatty, sugary, and salty foods. This doesn't mean you must eliminate them. You can still eat processed foods ecstatically, and *without* guilt. It can be very satisfying to occasionally enjoy your favorite high-fat meal or a rich dessert. But if you ate nothing but chocolate for two days straight, you would grow tired of it sooner or later, and you'd want healthier foods. It would lose its allure.

You can learn to really love eating a variety of healthy food. Besides tasting delicious, eating high quality foods will make you feel better. A well-balanced diet provides the nutrients you need to enhance your mood and energy levels.

Remember, ideally, you will eat when you are hungry, and then forget about eating until hunger strikes again. Food's place is to satisfy feelings of uncomfortable hunger so that you can get on with your life. Food should not be your greatest enjoyment in life. If it is, don't get mad at yourself. Rather, begin to fill your life with plenty of activities besides food that satisfy your heart and soul.

CHAPTER FIVE

You Deserve the Best

If you think of the standard American diet, it forms the acronym SAD. Sadly, this is fitting. The standard American diet is a sad way of eating. We are one of the richest countries in the world, yet many of us subsist on low-quality fuel, foods that increase our risk for dying early from diseases like diabetes, cancer, heart attack, and stroke, and also increase our chances for becoming overweight or obese. Here are just some of the foods that have very little nutritional value, yet that our nation as a whole consumes in excess:

- Drinks high in sugar like soda or drinks high in fat and sugar like some specialty coffee drinks, smoothies, and milkshakes
- High-fat fast food like pizza, hamburgers, and hot dogs
- Processed soups and boxed foods with lots of carbohydrates, salt, and often times fat (items like boxed rice, macaroni and cheese, and cups of noodles).
- Large servings of products like white noodles, white bread, white tortillas, white rice, and white rolls
- Deep fried foods like French fries, potato chips, and many appetizers
- Sweets like candy, cookies, baked goods, and ice cream
- Wine, beer, and mixed drinks

We've said it repeatedly, but we will say it again just to drive home the point, there's nothing wrong with having the foods listed above. However, for good health and weight loss, they shouldn't be a staple of your diet. Consume them in moderation, as an occasional treat. For example, if you really love ice cream, you could fit a small ice cream cone into your daily meal plan and still lose weight by eating mostly healthy foods and keeping your portions in check. But you probably would not lose weight if you had pepperoni pizza and a soda and ice cream all in one day unless you kept your portions of each very small.

If you acquired your dream car, you would surely take good care of it with good quality fuel and regular oil changes. Even so, a car can always be replaced. You can't trade in your body for a new one when it malfunctions. Yet many people force their bodies to continually run on low-grade fuel.

Do you believe your body is a premium machine that deserves the very finest? Maybe a better question to ask is: Do you believe you are so important and wonderful that *you* deserve only the best quality food? If your answer is yes, then you are ready for some tips that make caring for yourself easier. Maybe you are not actually going to climb a mountain. But every day, just to live, your body is relying on you to give it the nutrients it needs to function optimally.

Now it's time to shift gears. To begin, rather than considering all the foods you must reduce or eliminate, focus primarily on everything you are going to *include* in your diet. When it comes to losing weight, you're much more likely to keep it off if you make changes that add to your diet rather than subtract from it. If you think about all that you can't have, you're bound to feel deprived and eventually you'll overeat. However, if you focus on everything you *can* have, the changes you make will be easier.

What foods are the best for weight loss?

Just think plants! Rather than say, "I'm going to eliminate sugar," you could say, "I'm going to eat three fruit servings a day." If you are thinking about eliminating sugar, then sugar is your focus. It is the "bad" food that now has the power to make you fall halfway down the mountain if you sneak just a little taste. No food should have that kind of power. If you think you eat too many sweets, then think of a healthier way to get your fix. Fruit is a great low-calorie way to satisfy a sweet tooth.

If sweets aren't your thing, you might decide to add vegetables (not the bland old standby carrots and celery), but more interesting and tasty options. Try salads with all the fixings including some cheese or nuts and your favorite dressing, or roasted vegetables drizzled with oil and spices, or add veggies to your favorite ethnic dish. You don't need to become a rabbit to lose weight. The ability to prepare foods in flavorful ways is one of the great gifts of being human, and the foods you eat don't have to be low-calorie!

When you eat something with calories that tastes good, you'll more likely be satisfied and won't have to plow through a bunch of low-calorie items before you eventually get to the good stuff. Have the good stuff upfront, and you'll probably find you're less likely to overeat. As mentioned previously, if you deny yourself what you really want, you may consume thousands of tasteless calories in your attempt to feel gratified.

There are a hundred ways to lose weight and hundreds of books that will tell you what to eat. But none of those books know you personally—your preferences and struggles, your lifestyle and needs. This book allows you to figure out what will work for you—the master of your body. You get to make a plan to include all of the yummy, healthy foods that suit your taste buds, your schedule, and your way of life.

Eating healthy is a way you take care of your body. It is a way you show kindness and respect to yourself. You only have one body for life. As such, it is your most prized possession.

Build a Quality Base. A healthy diet consists of a variety of foods including whole grains, fruits, vegetables, lean protein, and either dairy products or another good source of calcium and vitamin D. You can combine these foods any way you like, according to your preferences.

In our society, huge portions have become the norm. But just because everybody's eating big doesn't mean it's healthy. On the contrary, it's killing us. So get out your measuring cups, a ruler, and maybe even a food scale so that you have an idea of how much to include.

The serving size you choose will depend on your current weight and height, so there is not one standard recommendation for everyone. The serving sizes listed below give you a good idea of how much to eat to allow your body to burn more calories over the course of a day than you take in. This means, of course, that you will lose weight. The key is to eat when you're hungry and stop when your hunger is gone, but before you are full, and definitely before you are stuffed. Here's a quick summary of what to eat most of the time. These serving sizes are recommended for the average, healthy adult. If you have special medical conditions, then these recommendations may not apply.

- **Eat 1 to 2 cups fruit per day.** Choose fruit without added sugar, and be sure to include at least one piece of raw fruit per day. One hundred percent juice counts as fruit but should be limited to no more than six ounces (3/4 cup) per day.

- **Eat at least 2 to 3 cups vegetables per day.** One hundred percent vegetable juice counts as a vegetable, but just as with fruit, aim to eat more whole vegetables for the added fiber. You can eat as many non-starchy vegetables as you like. Non-starchy vegetables are most vegetables and include: leafy greens, broccoli, carrots, peppers, tomatoes, etc., etc. Starchy vegetables include: potatoes, sweet potatoes, corn, peas, and squash. Limit starchy vegetables to one-half to one cup per day or use them in place of some of your grains.

- **Eat 4 to 7 ounces grains per day and make at least half of these whole grains.** Now, here's the kicker. This may sound like a lot. But it's NOT—at least compared to typical portion sizes. A pancake meal or two to three slices of pizza may contain all of the grains you need in a day. That's the bad news. The good news is that you *should* include grains (often referred to as carbohydrates). They aren't evil and won't turn directly into fat if you don't overdo it. Your body needs whole grains for energy, vitamins, minerals, and fiber.

  An ounce equals:
  - One-half cup **cooked** oatmeal, brown rice, whole-wheat pasta, quinoa, and the like. Note: serving sizes are *after* cooking
  - One slice of whole grain bread (this is your smaller sandwich bread that fits easily in a sandwich-size plastic bag)
  - A six-inch whole grain tortilla (the size of small corn tortillas)
  - One pancake (four and a half inches across)
  - Three-quarter to one cup of cold whole grain breakfast cereal (like shredded wheat or bran flakes)

- **Eat 5 to 9 ounces protein per day.** If you are less active, you can get away with less protein. If you are highly active you should eat a little more protein. You shouldn't need more than 9 ounces of protein per day unless you are working out vigorously for more than an hour daily. It's common knowledge that a 3-ounce piece of meat, poultry or fish is about the same length and width of a deck of cards. You can substitute the following types of protein for a meat serving:

o Three ounces tofu
o One-half cup of cooked dried beans and legumes (examples are navy, kidney, and refried beans, lentils, split peas)
o Two tablespoons nut butter
o Two eggs
o One cup of Greek yogurt or cottage cheese
o One-quarter cup of nuts or seeds (Nut butters and nuts don't have more protein, but should be limited to 2 tablespoons for butters and ¼ cup for nuts because they are high in calories and fat. The type of fat is mostly healthy, unsaturated fat, but eating too much can make it hard to lose weight.)

- **Eat two to three servings of dairy products or an alternative source of calcium and vitamin D.**
One serving equals:
  o 1 cup of 1%, skim, soy, almond, or rice milk
  o 1 cup of yogurt (soy versions included)
  o 1.5 ounces of cheese (soy versions included)

- **Eat healthier, unsaturated, fats.** Unsaturated fats are found in oils, fatty fish, nuts, seeds, and avocadoes. Less healthy saturated fats are found in fatty meats, butter, and regular or reduced-fat dairy products. Because all fat is high in calories, you don't want to overdo it on healthy fats. Just try to replace a good part of the saturated fat you are eating with healthy fats. You can consume unsaturated fats as part of the food you eat, for example, by eating a handful of nuts every day or a quarter of an avocado (again note the small portions). You can also add healthy fats by dipping your whole grain bread in a couple teaspoons of olive oil rather than using butter or margarine, or cooking with oils versus butter.

- **Flavor your food with herbs and spices.** Herbs and spices have many similar disease fighting nutrients that we find in fruits, vegetables, and other plant foods. If you are cutting back on fat and salt, they are an awesome way to add spunk to your meals.

- Check out the U.S. Department of Agriculture's www.choosemyplate.gov for more information. The recommendations on this website are based on research.

The Power of Plants. Besides watching how much you eat, good nutrition is vital to good health. Plant foods like whole grains, dried beans and other legumes, fruit, and vegetables are powerfully nutritious. They contain a variety of vitamins, minerals, phytochemicals, and fiber.

Phytochemicals are naturally occurring chemicals in plants that give them color and flavor. In humans, phytochemicals help to protect against diseases like heart disease, cancer, and diabetes. Some foods contain hundreds of phytochemicals and some very little. For example, there are as much as 75 percent more phytochemicals in a piece of whole wheat bread versus a piece of white bread. Likewise, a piece of whole fruit has more phytochemicals than an equivalent amount of juice.

Fiber is another key nutrient found in whole plant foods. It can help with weight loss, and can also help to lower your risk for diabetes, heart disease, and certain types of cancer.

Consider buying organic foods or foods with less pesticides and hormones used in their production. Researchers continually discover more and more chemicals added to our food or packaging that may be harmful to our health. Consume food that is less processed, meaning whole food that you cook yourself, to cut back on the amount of preservatives consumed.

Finally, get most of your nutrients from real food. Don't rely on vitamins to provide most of your nutrition. For example, instead of opting for some type of balanced nutrition bar for lunch that is heavily fortified with man-made vitamins, eat a meal that contains plenty of vegetables and at least one serving of lean protein, fruit, and whole grains. Nutrition bars often contain sugar and saturated fat, and you'll get more nutrition from a healthy meal of real food than the fortified supplements in the bar.

Leave Lots of Wiggle Room. We are going to be perfectly honest with you now. Although we (the authors) maintain a healthy weight and aim to feed our bodies well, we don't eat the exact foods and serving sizes above every single day. Some days we are *way* off track. But that's OKAY.

Nobody follows a flawless diet. It's impossible. You might have a day where you eat a donut for breakfast, a piece of pizza for lunch, and a burger for dinner. But you know what? If you control your portions, you can probably still lose weight eating these foods—or at least not gain. They aren't as nutritious, but one day won't make or break you. The key is to get your foothold back as soon as possible. Eat healthy most of the time.

A big part of weight loss depends on how many total calories you take in every day. Say you burn 1,850 calories a day to live and be active. If you take in only 1,600 calories per day, you will be in a 250 calorie deficit a day—meaning that your body had to burn 250 calories of fat or muscle stores in order to live. (To burn mostly fat, be sure to be physically active thirty to ninety minutes every day.) Over the course of a week, 250 calories adds up to 1,750 calories. Now, everyone's body is different and how much weight you lose will depend on your unique metabolism, but it's a fair guess that you would lose about one-half pound per week at a 250 calorie per day deficit.

The point is that calories COUNT! If you eat a quality base of foods, you can probably fit in a hundred to two hundred calories of junk and still watch the pounds disappear. If you want pizza for dinner, have a lighter lunch. If you want dessert, then eat less for dinner. If you want both pizza and dessert, then be sure and exercise more that day to offset the calories. Get the idea? Great! Eat, drink, and be merry!

CHAPTER SIX

When Food Means More than Air
Dealing with Overpowering Urges

An urge to eat when you aren't hungry can build gradually, or it can hit you like a sudden hurricane with a force so powerful you are helpless to stop it. You may feel completely out of control as you surrender to your desire to eat. Afterward, you may wonder what happened, and how so much damage could have occurred in such a short amount of time.

In order to get to the point where your urges for food no longer have this kind of power, you need to understand the process of craving, beginning with how you are provoked. Urges to eat can arise from both internal and external factors.

Internal factors that arouse cravings include thoughts about food or certain feelings, such as boredom, sadness, or even happiness. Remembering your grandmother fondly could lead to thoughts of her chocolate cake with fudge frosting, and the craving has begun.

External factors that arouse cravings include the smell or sight of certain foods or watching others eat. Driving by a restaurant you like, looking at recipes, television commercials, or cooking shows can all activate a craving for food.

The Mind Game. Let's pretend that you love chocolate. But you normally deny yourself chocolate for fear that you will overdo it. Imagine walking into a room with your very favorite chocolate wrapped in red foil hearts in a basket on the table. You suddenly get a strong urge to eat the chocolate.

What happens next depends on your frame of mind.

You might eat the chocolate at once without stopping to decide if it's the best choice for you. If you don't have a weight problem or problems with overeating, you might eat a piece or two or three with no guilt, feel satisfied, and get on with life. If you do have problems with your weight or overeating, you will likely feel very guilty after eating the chocolate. You might wake up while eating it, and ask yourself, "What am I doing?" Or maybe after you finish off the basket of chocolate you'll ask, "Why did I have to eat all that? *Why?*" This can lead to more overeating, which we will discuss in the next section.

You might deliberate over whether to eat the chocolate. Your mind plays the game: *To Eat or Not to Eat.* You see the chocolate and your thinking mind tells you that you can't have it. But another part of your mind begins to focus on the experience of the chocolate. You think about how good it will smell, how rich it will taste, and how creamy it will feel in your mouth. This craving business is really a very sensual process. If you are all alone, the chocolate may be even more difficult to resist. Nobody is there to stop you from taking what you want.

At this point, you may begin to rationalize your desire. "I'll just have one. It's no big deal. One piece of chocolate won't hurt."

But then again, maybe a part of you is really resolved **not** to eat the chocolate. So you hesitate. You pick it up. You hold it. You put it back. You pick it up again. Your mind is split into two factions. Maybe it only takes a few seconds, but your thoughts are firing rapidly from both sides.

Part of you says: "Just eat it. You deserve a treat. You need a pick-me-up. This is your only pleasure. You've had it rough. Give yourself a break. It'll be so good. You can't deny it. It's too tempting. You'll never eat something this good again. You'll make up for it tomorrow. You have to have it. You need it more than air!"

Another part says: "You really don't need it. You're not hungry. Walk away. Go exercise. Call a friend. Find something else to do. You have to resist. It'll make you gain weight. You'll regret it later."

If you make the decision to indulge, you feel great anticipation at the thought that you are about to enjoy the chocolate. You may become very excited—on a high—and your senses become aroused by your rebellion. You are about to break your rules and engage in a forbidden act. Your heart rate speeds up. Your world narrows. All you can think about is you and your desire.

The craving gains strength, like a snowball rolling down a hill getting bigger and bigger. At some point, the snowball knocks you over.

Giving Into the Imagined Ecstasy. You quickly remove the chocolate from the wrapper and indulge. As you do so, you experience a sudden, welcoming release. You no longer have to resist. Your mind is no longer in so much tension about indulging or not indulging. You have succumbed. The chocolate is pure ecstasy. Or maybe it's not. Maybe it doesn't even taste as good as you believed it would. You feel better for an instant, and then quickly begin to feel worse.

You start to think that you have broken down, that you have not kept your commitment to yourself, and that you have failed.

With all of this banter in your mind about how you shouldn't be eating, or how you blew it, it's impossible to fully enjoy the chocolate. Rather than really being present to notice all of those wonderful qualities of the chocolate you had dreamed about before popping it into your mouth, you are stuck in your thoughts, missing out on the actual experience.

If you truly feel bad, then you might tell yourself, "Well, I just blew it. I may as well keep going and polish off the basket. I'll get back on track tomorrow." This is where you turn a craving into a problem. Giving into one piece of chocolate is not a big deal. It equates to 100 or 200 calories. This amount of calories from chocolate fits into any healthy weight loss plan. But when you criticize yourself and believe you've failed by eating one piece of chocolate, that one piece often turns into ten or twenty pieces (in other words, thousands of calories).

After overeating on the chocolate, you likely feel disgusted with yourself. You wonder why you can't just get it together. You make promises to yourself that you'll have better willpower the next time. You will no longer succumb to temptation. Maybe you follow a strict diet plan. Maybe you get some exercise. You do well for a few hours, a few days, or even a few weeks. But then, something activates your craving again.

Chocolate sings your name, calling to you like a long lost friend. An overwhelming desire and excitement take hold as you consider eating the chocolate, your forbidden fruit. The urge to eat builds and the process repeats itself.

Become a Spectator. Start to watch your mind games. The human mind is a genius at justifying reasons why we should overeat. The mind is very good at rationalizing and justifying behaviors. Notice what commonly activates your urges to eat. Notice what thoughts arise for you. Notice the feelings. Notice the boxing match in your head, with part of you fighting to eat, and part of you fighting to avoid eating.

Do your urges win every single time? Are you sometimes able to overcome your urges and not act on them? If so, how do you do this? How can you do it more often?

You don't need to be taken over by your urges, but nor do you need to always resist. The key is to find a balance between the two. You can acknowledge and satisfy your cravings without going overboard and wrecking your health or weight loss goals.

When you eat, don't project yourself into the future with thoughts about how you will have to work off every last calorie. Don't project yourself into the past by saying, "I have always failed. I've never had self-control."

With practice, you can begin to notice signs that an urge to eat is building within you and learn to prevent a craving from overwhelming you. No longer a victim, you will be in charge of making your own weather. You will not suffer the storms that result from repeatedly allowing cravings to dominate your life.

If you decide to give into your craving, don't worry about it. Instead, be with your food and in your senses. Taste the food and fully enjoy it. Relish in it. You may enjoy the food more this way. Or, when you really taste it, you may find that it's not even as good as you thought.

As you eat, watch judgmental thoughts about your behavior drift past without completely believing them or identifying with them. Then allow yourself to make a new choice.

Check in with your stomach as you eat. How does it feel? What sensations do you notice? Do you feel empty? Or full? Are you neither empty nor full? Are you getting full?

Alternative Delights. There are many other wonderful sensory experiences in life besides eating. In fact, the entire body is a sensory delight, offering you the gift of sight, taste, touch, smell, and hearing.

Discovering other joys can help shift your focus away from food. You can expand your sources of delight to a whole host of experiences: You can feast with your eyes at a beautiful sunrise; you can inhale sharply the fresh, crisp morning air; you can smell the delightful aroma of fresh cut flowers; and you can feel the warmth and pressure of a shower massager, just to name a few of the many ways to engage your senses.

What brings you pleasure? Here are some activities to engage your senses. Notice that some of the activities engage more than one sense at a time. Note the ones you like, and also add any other activities you can think of.

Sight:

- Go outside and watch the clouds (or view them from a window)
- Take a scenic drive
- Go for a walk or hike in nature
- View animals at a pet store
- Go to an art gallery
- Look at artistic magazines

Touch:

- Bask in the sun (you can wear sunscreen) and enjoy the warmth
- Take a hot bath with bath salts
- Get a massage
- Give yourself a facial
- Have sex with a significant other (someone you love)

Smell:

- Light a candle and enjoy the scent along with the sight of the dancing flame
- Wear a perfume you like

- Apply scented lotion or lip balm
- Go outside and breathe in the scent of fresh air
- Keep a vase of fresh flowers at home or work

Hearing:
- Play music you enjoy
- Sing or learn to sing
- Sit by the ocean or by a river or creek and listen to the water flow
- Walk through a park and listen to the shouts of joy from young children
- Turn on the radio or TV just for background noise

Taste:
- Make herbal tea or coffee and drink it without added sugar. Notice the complex flavors
- Chew a stick of gum
- Eat one square of chocolate very slowly, focusing intently on the taste
- Suck on a lemon or lime wedge
- Chew on a flavored toothpick

CHAPTER SEVEN

Playtime

What is playtime? Physical activity, of course. You may not agree. In fact, you may consider physical activity to be torture, not play. Society teaches that exercise is punishment and food is reward. Music students are taught the mnemonic "Every Good Boy Deserves Fudge" to recall the notes on the treble clef (EGBDF). We have the idea that when we are good, we deserve to reward ourselves with food. When we are bad, we think of the army drill sergeant commanding, "Drop and give me twenty!"

You have probably heard somebody say, "I have to go exercise after eating all that!" Maybe you've said it yourself. But it's doubtful you've heard someone say, "I want to go run around at the park for an hour, so I guess I have to eat an ice cream cone." This would mean that food would be a punishment, exercise a reward.

Personally, Holly used to view exercise as the penance she paid for eating so much. Since she binge ate, she would often think of exercise in terms of calories burned. She'd say to herself, "I just ate 2,000 calories in one setting so I need to burn at least 1,500 of those calories." She'd go to the gym and ride the bike, followed by the elliptical, the treadmill, and finally, the weights. All of this took a total of two miserable hours. Looking back, Holly can see it was two hours at a time that she wasted. She rarely enjoyed herself, and she'd often end up going home and overeating just to do it all again.

After these marathon workouts, Holly felt completely exhausted. And she was always getting sick. Her body wasn't healthy despite all of the physical activity. She grew to hate exercise, and began alternating through periods of time when she forced herself to do it and periods of time when she barely moved at all.

Holly was out of touch with her body's needs. She didn't realize that her body did want to move daily, that it felt good to move. But her body did not enjoy or respond well to the extreme exercise bouts she often put it through. She needed to find a balance. She also needed to find exercise that was fun.

Fast-forward twenty years, and Holly loves exercise. It truly is her playtime. Sometimes she works out alone by taking a jog outside or doing an exercise DVD, but often she works out with friends and family. Together with the people she loves, she skis, hikes, mountain bikes, jogs, and rides a dirt-jump bike on a pump track (even though she's now a forty year-old woman).

The truth is that exercise can be very rewarding. The human body was made to move. Our ancestors moved constantly in order to survive. Today, we sit most of the day, with intermittent movement. We barely have to move at all and can still get our needs met. However, this leaves us with out-of-shape bodies that don't feel good.

In working with people who are in pain or injured and believe they can't exercise, Holly has seen over and over that once they begin to exercise, their pain lessens. Often it is not their body holding them back, but their mind. They believe they can't do half of what they are capable of doing. Sure, they may not be able to do as much activity as they once could. But they can do a lot more than they actually think they can. As injured persons increase their movement, their injury usually becomes less severe. Their mental state improves. They feel better and better. They want to do more and more movement. Exercise becomes a habit.

The U.S. Department of Health and Human Services *Physical Activity Guidelines for Americans* say that people need at least 150 minutes of activity a week for good health. This can be broken down however you like. You could choose to do a half-hour of exercise, five days a week, or just over twenty minutes a day. You might also do two one-hour sessions and one 30-minute session per week.

This really isn't a lot of exercise. Our ancestors walked an average of ten miles a day, and we know that for weight loss, more may be needed—up to

60 to 90 minutes of activity a day. This includes any kind of movement where you're raising your heart rate and body temperature.

Did you know that you can break up your exercise bouts into ten-minute sessions and still get the same health and weight loss benefits? So you might do ten minutes of yoga in the morning, go for a ten minute walk at noon, and ride the bike for ten minutes in the evening to get your 30 minutes of activity in per day.

The body craves movement. Think back to when you were a kid. What kind of physical activity did you like? Whether it's dancing, kickboxing, karate, tennis, basketball, swimming, powerlifting, golfing, or mountaineering, the beauty of human beings are that we are all different. What one person loves another may deplore. Get creative. You can find an activity that you love—or at least one you don't detest.

Try to take five to ten minutes every hour or two to move around. Or schedule activity like you would an appointment, and keep the appointment. Make it a priority in your life.

In this book, we have introduced you to setting YOUR Action Goals. We haven't told you what to do or how to do it. That is because you are the master of you. Only you know the changes to your eating habits or exercise regimen that will work. So figure out what does it for you, and commit to giving it all you've got. We are honored that you spent this time with us. This is just the start of a happier, thinner you!

Quick Reminders to Help you Succeed with your Action Goals

- Remember that your outcome (weight loss) is not your goal.
- Make your goal something you can do today.
- Tell others about your goals, share what you learn along the way, and talk about your success.
- Make goals and exercise fun. It doesn't have to be grueling.
- Find a trigger to remind you of your goals.
- Don't be judgmental about yourself or what you do.
- Take one step at a time and don't overwhelm yourself.
- Stay positive.
- Take a time out.
- Ask how the food you are eating will affect your body?
- Eat mindfully – slow down and notice the flavors of the food as you eat.
- Keep tempting foods out of sight or possibly out of the house.
- Keep plenty of healthy foods that you like on hand.
- Try not to sneak food. If you really want it, eat it openly.
- Eat when you are hungry (don't get overly hungry).
- Commit to the fact that you are not on a temporary diet.
- Just because you mess up, the whole day is not ruined. Just get back on track.
- Remember there are no bad foods.
- Find other ways to experience pleasure besides food.
- Try to move a little bit every day. Any physical activity is better than nothing.
- Take the time for you. Make yourself a priority!

Desired Outcome: _____

Date:_____

_____

Specific Action:_____

_____

When will you start:_____

What Days and Times?_____

_____

How will you accomplish?_____

_____

What do you need?_____

_____

How will you make it fun?_____

_____

_____

Who do you tell?_____

_____

What will get in your way?_____

_____

How will you overcome challenges?_____

_____

_____

Week 1

Make sure your goal is something you can do today, an action not an outcome.

Date:_____

What were you able to accomplish?_____

_____

_____

_____

Learning moments, what did you learn?_____

_____

_____

_____

What will you do different, if anything?_____

_____

_____

What did others say about your accomplishments?_____

_____

_____

How do you feel about your accomplishments?_____

_____

_____

Your new modified goal, if you changed it:_____

_____

_____

New Goals

Date:_____

Specific Action:_____
_____

When will you start:_____

What Days and Times?_____
_____

How will you accomplish?_____
_____

What do you need?_____
_____

How will you make it fun?_____
_____
_____

What will get in your way?_____

_____

How will you overcome challenges?_____
_____

_____

What successes have you had so far?_____
_____

_____

New Goals

Date:_____

Specific Action:_____

_____

When will you start:_____

What Days and Times?_____

_____

How will you accomplish?_____

_____

What do you need?_____

_____

How will you make it fun?_____

_____

_____

What will get in your way?_____

_____

How will you overcome challenges?_____

_____

_____

What successes have you had so far?_____

_____

_____

Week 2

It's important to involve others. Take the time to share your successes or talk about lessons learned. They may even come up with more great ideas.

Date:_____

What were you able to accomplish?_____

_____

_____

_____

Learning moments, what did you learn?_____

_____

_____

_____

What will you do different, if anything?_____

_____

_____

What did others say about your accomplishments?_____

_____

_____

How do you feel about your accomplishments?_____

_____

_____

Your new modified goal, if you changed it:_____

_____

_____

New Goals

Date:_____

Specific Action:_____
_____

When will you start:_____

What Days and Times?_____

_____

How will you accomplish?_____

_____

What do you need?_____

_____

How will you make it fun?_____

_____

_____

What will get in your way?_____

_____

How will you overcome challenges?_____

_____

_____

What successes have you had so far?_____

_____

_____

New Goals

Date:_____

Specific Action:_____
_____

When will you start:_____

What Days and Times?_____
_____

How will you accomplish?_____
_____

What do you need?_____
_____

How will you make it fun?_____
_____
_____

What will get in your way?_____
_____

How will you overcome challenges?_____
_____
_____

What successes have you had so far?_____
_____
_____

Week 3

Remember, don't judge yourself.

Date:_____

What were you able to accomplish?_____

_____

_____

_____

Learning moments, what did you learn?_____

_____

_____

_____

What will you do different, if anything?_____

_____

_____

What did others say about your accomplishments?_____

_____

_____

How do you feel about your accomplishments?_____

_____

_____

Your new modified goal, if you changed it:_____

_____

_____

New Goals

Date:_____

Specific Action:_____
_____

When will you start:_____

What Days and Times?_____
_____

How will you accomplish?_____
_____

What do you need?_____
_____

How will you make it fun?_____
_____
_____

What will get in your way?_____
_____

How will you overcome challenges?_____
_____
_____

What successes have you had so far?_____
_____
_____

New Goals

Date:_____

Specific Action:_____
_____

When will you start:_____

What Days and Times?_____
_____

How will you accomplish?_____
_____

What do you need?_____
_____

How will you make it fun?_____
_____
_____

What will get in your way?_____
_____

How will you overcome challenges?_____
_____
_____

What successes have you had so far?_____
_____
_____

Week 4

Think of the tortoise and the hair and take one step at a time.

Date:_____

What were you able to accomplish?_____

_____

_____

_____

_____

Learning moments, what did you learn?_____

_____

_____

_____

What will you do different, if anything?_____

_____

_____

What did others say about your accomplishments?_____

_____

_____

How do you feel about your accomplishments?_____

_____

_____

Your new modified goal, if you changed it:_____

_____

_____

New Goals

Date:_____

Specific Action:_____

_____

When will you start:_____

What Days and Times?_____

_____

How will you accomplish?_____

_____

What do you need?_____

_____

How will you make it fun?_____

_____

_____

What will get in your way?_____

_____

How will you overcome challenges?_____

_____

_____

What successes have you had so far?_____

_____

_____

New Goals

Date:_____

Specific Action:_____
_____

When will you start:_____

What Days and Times?_____
_____

How will you accomplish?_____
_____

What do you need?_____
_____

How will you make it fun?_____
_____
_____

What will get in your way?_____
_____

How will you overcome challenges?_____
_____
_____

What successes have you had so far?_____
_____
_____

Week 5

Do you have to drag yourself to get your goal done? If so, can you think of a way to make it more fun?

Date:_____

What were you able to accomplish?_____

_____

_____

_____

Learning moments, what did you learn?_____

_____

_____

_____

What will you do different, if anything?_____

_____

_____

What did others say about your accomplishments?____

_____

_____

How do you feel about your accomplishments?_____

_____

_____

Your new modified goal, if you changed it:_____

_____

_____

New Goals

Date:_____

Specific Action:_____

_____

When will you start:_____

What Days and Times?_____

_____

How will you accomplish?_____

_____

What do you need?_____

_____

How will you make it fun?_____

_____

_____

What will get in your way?_____

_____

How will you overcome challenges?_____

_____

_____

What successes have you had so far?_____

_____

_____

New Goals

Date:_____

Specific Action:_____
_____

When will you start:_____

What Days and Times?_____
_____

How will you accomplish?_____
_____

What do you need?_____
_____

How will you make it fun?_____
_____
_____

What will get in your way?_____
_____

How will you overcome challenges?_____
_____

What successes have you had so far?_____
_____
_____

Week 6

When you don't succeed, make sure to look at it as a learning moment, not as a failure.

Date:_____

What were you able to accomplish?_____
_____
_____
_____
_____

Learning moments, what did you learn?_____
_____
_____
_____

What will you do different, if anything?_____
_____
_____

What did others say about your accomplishments?____
_____
_____

How do you feel about your accomplishments?_____
_____
_____

Your new modified goal, if you changed it:_____
_____
_____

New Goals

Date:_____

Specific Action:_____
_____

When will you start:_____

What Days and Times?_____
_____

How will you accomplish?_____
_____

What do you need?_____
_____

How will you make it fun?_____
_____
_____

What will get in your way?_____
_____

How will you overcome challenges?_____
_____
_____

What successes have you had so far?_____
_____
_____

New Goals

Date:_____

Specific Action:_____
_____

When will you start:_____

What Days and Times?_____
_____

How will you accomplish?_____
_____

What do you need?_____
_____

How will you make it fun?_____
_____
_____

What will get in your way?_____
_____

How will you overcome challenges?_____
_____
_____

What successes have you had so far?_____
_____
_____

Week 7

Eat mindfully, noticing why you are eating, whether or not you are hungry, how the food will affect your body, and how it tastes.

Date:_____

What were you able to accomplish?_____

_____

_____

_____

_____

Learning moments, what did you learn?_____

_____

_____

_____

What will you do different, if anything?_____

_____

_____

What did others say about your accomplishments?_____

_____

_____

How do you feel about your accomplishments?_____

_____

_____

Your new modified goal, if you changed it:_____

_____

_____

New Goals

Date:_____

Specific Action:_____
_____

When will you start:_____

What Days and Times?_____
_____

How will you accomplish?_____
_____

What do you need?_____
_____

How will you make it fun?_____
_____
_____

What will get in your way?_____
_____

How will you overcome challenges?_____
_____
_____

What successes have you had so far?_____
_____
_____

New Goals

Date:_____

Specific Action:_____
_____

When will you start:_____

What Days and Times?_____
_____

How will you accomplish?_____
_____

What do you need?_____
_____

How will you make it fun?_____
_____
_____

What will get in your way?_____
_____

How will you overcome challenges?_____
_____
_____

What successes have you had so far?_____
_____
_____

Week 8

Set yourself up for success. Keep tempting foods out of sight and plenty of healthy foods that you enjoy on hand.

Date:_____

What were you able to accomplish?_____

_____

_____

_____

Learning moments, what did you learn?_____

_____

_____

_____

What will you do different, if anything?_____

_____

_____

What did others say about your accomplishments?____

_____

_____

How do you feel about your accomplishments?_____

_____

_____

Your new modified goal, if you changed it:_____

_____

_____

New Goals

Date:_____

Specific Action:_____
_____

When will you start:_____

What Days and Times?_____
_____

How will you accomplish?_____
_____

What do you need?_____
_____

How will you make it fun?_____
_____
_____

What will get in your way?_____
_____

How will you overcome challenges?_____
_____
_____

What successes have you had so far?_____
_____
_____

New Goals

Date:_____

Specific Action:_____
_____

When will you start:_____

What Days and Times?_____
_____

How will you accomplish?_____
_____

What do you need?_____
_____

How will you make it fun?_____
_____
_____

What will get in your way?_____
_____

How will you overcome challenges?_____
_____
_____

What successes have you had so far?_____
_____
_____

Week 9

Try not to sneak food. Eat openly and enjoy it regardless of what other people may think of your eating choices.

Date:_____

What were you able to accomplish?_____

_____

_____

_____

_____

Learning moments, what did you learn?_____

_____

_____

_____

What will you do different, if anything?_____

_____

_____

What did others say about your accomplishments?____

_____

_____

How do you feel about your accomplishments?_____

_____

_____

Your new modified goal, if you changed it:_____

_____

_____

New Goals

Date:_____

Specific Action:_____
_____

When will you start:_____

What Days and Times?_____
_____

How will you accomplish?_____
_____

What do you need?_____
_____

How will you make it fun?_____
_____
_____

What will get in your way?_____
_____

How will you overcome challenges?_____
_____
_____

What successes have you had so far?_____
_____
_____

New Goals

Date:_____

Specific Action:_____

_____

When will you start:_____

What Days and Times?_____

_____

How will you accomplish?_____

_____

What do you need?_____

_____

How will you make it fun?_____

_____

_____

What will get in your way?_____

_____

How will you overcome challenges?_____

_____

_____

What successes have you had so far?_____

_____

_____

Week 10

Remember that you can eat anything you want. There are no bad foods. Adopt an overall healthy way of eating that makes room for your favorite foods.

Date:_____

What were you able to accomplish?_____

_____

_____

_____

Learning moments, what did you learn?_____

_____

_____

_____

What will you do different, if anything?_____

_____

_____

What did others say about your accomplishments?_____

_____

_____

How do you feel about your accomplishments?_____

_____

_____

Your new modified goal, if you changed it:_____

_____

_____

New Goals

Date:_____

Specific Action:_____
_____

When will you start:_____

What Days and Times?_____
_____

How will you accomplish?_____
_____

What do you need?_____
_____

How will you make it fun?_____
_____
_____

What will get in your way?_____
_____

How will you overcome challenges?_____
_____
_____

What successes have you had so far?_____
_____
_____

New Goals

Date:_____

Specific Action:_____

_____

When will you start:_____

What Days and Times?_____

_____

How will you accomplish?_____

_____

What do you need?_____

_____

How will you make it fun?_____

_____

_____

What will get in your way?_____

_____

How will you overcome challenges?_____

_____

_____

What successes have you had so far?_____

_____

_____

Week 11

If you end up overeating, forgive yourself immediately and get back on track making healthy choices right away.

Date:_____

What were you able to accomplish?_____

_____

_____

_____

_____

Learning moments, what did you learn?_____

_____

_____

_____

What will you do different, if anything?_____

_____

_____

What did others say about your accomplishments?____

_____

_____

How do you feel about your accomplishments?_____

_____

_____

Your new modified goal, if you changed it:_____

_____

_____

New Goals

Date:_____

Specific Action:_____
_____

When will you start:_____

What Days and Times?_____
_____

How will you accomplish?_____
_____

What do you need?_____
_____

How will you make it fun?_____
_____
_____

What will get in your way?_____
_____

How will you overcome challenges?_____
_____
_____

What successes have you had so far?_____
_____
_____

New Goals

Date:_____

Specific Action:_____
_____

When will you start:_____

What Days and Times?_____
_____

How will you accomplish?_____
_____

What do you need?_____
_____

How will you make it fun?_____
_____
_____

What will get in your way?_____
_____

How will you overcome challenges?_____
_____

What successes have you had so far?_____
_____
_____

Week 12

Try to move your body at least a little bit every day. Make a list of all the ways you can be active over the next week and commit to doing the activities.

Date:_____

What were you able to accomplish?_____

_____

_____

_____

_____

Learning moments, what did you learn?_____

_____

_____

_____

What will you do different, if anything?_____

_____

_____

What did others say about your accomplishments?____

_____

_____

How do you feel about your accomplishments?_____

_____

_____

Your new modified goal, if you changed it:_____

_____

_____

New Goals

Date:_____

Specific Action:_____
_____

When will you start:_____

What Days and Times?_____
_____

How will you accomplish?_____
_____

What do you need?_____
_____

How will you make it fun?_____
_____
_____

What will get in your way?_____
_____

How will you overcome challenges?_____
_____
_____

What successes have you had so far?_____
_____
_____

New Goals

Date:_____

Specific Action:_____

_____

When will you start:_____

What Days and Times?_____

_____

How will you accomplish?_____

_____

What do you need?_____

_____

How will you make it fun?_____

_____

_____

What will get in your way?_____

_____

How will you overcome challenges?_____

_____

_____

What successes have you had so far?_____

_____

_____

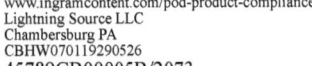